Praise for, Your Life is Medicine: Ayurveda for Yogis

I just finished the last page of Your Life Is Medicine. As I put it down beside me, I was truly sad it was finished. It's been my trusted companion for the past weeks. It made me feel safe and grounded on so many occasions, especially when I felt anxy and while battling my little devil. I finished most evenings and started many mornings with it in my hands. I laughed and went AHA! a hundred times and can honestly say it has been the most enlightening read for me since The Untethered Soul. Only just now when I put it down, I fully got why the author chose that particular picture for the cover. That little thing called balance! Made me smile so much. I suspect this won't be the last book of Ms. Schneider I read. Watch this space.

—Amazon customer

This book is AMAZING. The opening letter and story were enough to grip me and I fell in love with it immediately. The way the writer says and explains everything is so digestible and she is so humble! Ayurveda is one of the world's oldest medical systems designed to help prevent dis-ease and bring/keep your body/mind/spirit in balance. As a yoga teacher and one who LOVES and sees how important Ayurveda is for a healthy life I am so happy, she wrote this book. I have researched, studied and read a lot on Ayurveda. I have taken advanced Ayurveda courses and seen a couple of Ayurvedic Practitioners, assisted with Ayurvedic massages (as a Massage Therapist) and most importantly (as much as I can) I LIVE an Ayurvedic life. AND NOW Kristen puts it so simply WHY I do it and WHY it works and HOW to make it work for you. I have had the pleasure of meeting this wonderful author, Ayurvedic Practitioner and Yoga teacher, and she is as humble and sweet as she sounds from her book. I could go on and on!! I HIGHLY recommend this healing book to everyone!

—Amazon Customer

I finished this book in under a week, reading half of it the first night and immediately began implementing some of the simple changes into my diet and routine. As a mental health therapist I can't emphasize the importance of self-care enough, but this book challenged me to take my own self-care to a new level. It is a very helpful book and I recommend it to whoever will listen as it is written so that anyone can understand it. I read a lot of books, and practice yoga and vedic astrology, so much of the information and concepts were familiar but the author pulled it all together and presented it in a way that really "clicked" something inside for me. My diet has been an ongoing point of frustration because I'm not a dieter. I never had to worry before since getting older I have been trying to find a way of eating that works for me. Since implementing many of the suggestions in the book, I feel great already and I have been having a really fun time doing it. I think this is a wonderful holistic presentation of the material and a wonderful contribution to the topic of "self-care".

—Amazon Customer

This is not a book, but a companion, not to be read and shelved but to accompany anyone who is striving for balanced and harmony in their life. I love the kindness and enthusiasm in the author's voice. She is not condemning me for my past mistakes and lifestyle choices. Instead, she offers encouragement and camaraderie with a voice that says, 'trust me, I've been there, I've tried those paths too and they didn't work for me either, but this one has and I am so excited to share it with you,' followed by clear and inviting steps to do just that. I especially enjoyed the personal stories of the author's own journey in discovering the world of Ayurveda and in doing so finding balance and healing for her own body. Bravo!

—Amazon Customer

This book is truly incredibly. If you have been searching for Ayurveda answers in a clean, concise, and well-organized way in a truly authentic, caring, and personal voice...LOOK NO FURTHER. Ms. Schneider has created a resource for the novice and master alike. Move at your pace. Allow yourself to absorb the philosophy. Making small transitions will make you a believer in this system.

—Amazon Customer

YOUR LIFE *is* MEDICINE

Ayurveda for Yogis

SECOND EDITION

KRISTEN LILLIAN SCHNEIDER

First Printing: 2019
ISBN 978-1-64606-492-2

www.wellblends.com

Cover and Book Interior Design by: Najdan Mancic, Iskon Design
Author's Portraits by: Chloe Clifton

Second Edition…NEW MATERIAL!

- Marma Points and Face Massage
- Tongue Diagnostics
- New Poetry
- How Doshas influence our dreams, spending habits, and careers
- Essential Oils for the Doshas
- New Recipes
- Home Remedies for Common Imbalances

Contents

PART II: Nutriton And Healing

"Ayurveda treatment begins with the narrative of the patient. It is the function of the Practitioner to direct people towards happiness. The Declaration of Independence declares our basic right to the pursuit of happiness. But I disagree—happiness is not something we achieve by pursuing. We find happiness by pursuing other things…our purpose. When we find our purpose, we achieve healing."

—Gerard Buffo

Dean of Kripalu School of Ayurveda

Letter from your Author...

THIS BOOK WAS originally published just over three years ago. At the time of first writing this book I had been practicing yoga for seven years, and Ayurveda for five. I had completed Ayurveda school and earned accreditation as a Board Certified Ayurveda Practitioner. I was three years into owning a small Ayurveda clinic in Orlando, Florida, where I had already met with about five hundred clients. I had experiential data on how Ayurveda had transformed my personal life, and I was watching it do the same for others right before my eyes. Early into my practice, patterns of common themes and shared imbalances become obvious to me. The majority of my clients seemed stress, inflamed, and anxious. Most of us had battled with food and body image, and a hard time juggling all the balls in our life. Self-care had taken a backseat in the lives of most of the people I saw. And having enough time to work and sleep, let alone cook healthy meals and exercise seemed to be a ubiquitous challenge. My motivation for publishing *Your Life is Medicine: Ayurveda for Yogis* was simple. I wanted to impart Ayurveda's simple, yet profound wisdom onto my clients and students. I wanted to distill the principles that can seem complicated at first glance. My goal was to curate the core message of Ayurveda, which is to return to your True Nature in a way that was both approachable and applicable. I think it was a success! Now, just over three years and 3,000 copies sold later; I have decided to reformat that book and create a second addition that carries an even more salient message and added tools. The original book was used for trainings and workshops. In such, it was large and looked more like a text book. The aesthetic of the larger book might have seemed intimidating for people who did not wish to "study" Ayurveda, or be students of the practice; but more so, just wanted to bring the concepts directly into their lives. I appreciate that, and that's why this book is more compact. You can toss it in your purse and read it at the park while your kids are playing. You can bring it with you and reference it as you stroll through the aisles at the grocery store, and you can keep it by your bedside to read at your leisure at night. The subtitle of this book is *Ayurveda for Yogis*. But this book is in no way exclusively for people who practice yoga. This book is for everyone! Yoga was my gateway into Ayurveda. I teach classes and trainings all over the world. As an avid student and practitioner of yoga—I think like a yogi. I see the world through the lens of largely Eastern philosophies. My story that of a woman who practices yoga. That is my experience, and I find it most authentic to share from experience. So that is why it's titled *Ayurveda for Yogis*. But I am not just a yogi. I am a daughter, a sister, a partner, an entrepreneur, an American, a modern woman, a students, a teacher, and sometimes, just like you—overwhelmed, exhausted, and seeking answers. This book is written as a source of inspiration, clarity, and ease. From my heart to yours, this book was written for you.

PART 1

Dosha Balancing Lifestyle

"Travel light, live light, spread light, be the light."

—Yogi Bhajan

INTRODUCTION

Opening Story...

YOU HAVE TASTED, experienced and embodied the benefits of yoga. If you are anything like me, on any given day you have been tired, wound up, anxious or stressed out as your ten toes made their way onto the yoga mat. Thanks to the generous and ineffable laws of the practice, you stepped off the mat just moments later feeling light, energized, calm, and at peace. You are well aware of how breath, movement, awareness, and intention meet time and space to transform your mood, day and even your life. You certainly have your own unique and inspiring story of how yoga has changed your life. Thank goodness for that. Thank goodness for yoga, and thank goodness for you. I solute you for having the curiosity, willingness, and commitment to improving your life. And by the contagious effects of energy, improving the lives of the people around you. No matter how your story began, fast forward and you find yourself here with this book in your hand. Perhaps you have the same intrigued, nervous, or trusting feeling in your heart as you did the day you entered your first yoga class. There is a deep knowingness that something is about to shift. I'm grateful you are here ready to explore, share, create, and shift. Wether we know each other by name or not, we share a connection. We share similar ideals, to love and be loved in return. We all do our best to treat ourselves with compassion and love, and to treat others with the same sentiment. We want to understand ourselves, feel vibrant, healthy, and happy. We are so much more alike than we are different. I'd like to introduce you to Ayurveda, the sister science of yoga. An approach to life that amalgamates science and spirituality. Ayurveda gives us the tools to celebrate our unity and nourish our individuality. Ayurveda is built on the premise that self-knowledge leads to self-healing. Ayurveda will be the perfect consort to your yoga practice. The heartbeat of Ayurveda is self-care. The way we care for ourselves and treat ourselves is the impetus for our individual health and the health of the planet. The process of learning Ayurveda, sharing the tools and even writing this book have enhanced my life in ways I would have never predicted or imagined. Like yoga, the science in infinite. The practice is continuously evolving, and we will all—always be students.

> *"The body is your temple. Keep it pure and clean for the soul to reside in."*
>
> **—B.K.S. Iyengar**

I was twenty-three years old when I stepped off the airplane for my first adventure in India. The plan was to take a six week long yoga course. As fate would have it, I ended up staying six months and that was just the start of the journey. I was living in a small town called Rishikesh. This town was known as the yoga mecca of the world. I found ashrams or spiritual communities, temples, and yoga schools galore. People walked down the streets draped in saffron robes and prayer beads. The aroma in the streets was a wafting cacophony of curry and cow manure, combined with the palpable aura of incense. You could not walk more than a few steps without passing beggars pleading for money, saints blessings your path, yogis standing on their heads, and shop owners trying to sell you trinkets. I stayed in an ashram with a couple girlfriends I met while living in China, teaching English the year prior. Oddly enough, I originally learned yoga in China. I did not speak Mandarin, so I learned purely off observation, trial, and plenty of error. My friends Naomi and Kathy, whom I practiced with in China decided they too loved yoga enough to fly to India and take a proper course. We arrived in January. It was freezing. Our accommodations had no heat or running water. The electricity was spotty and never functioned after 8am.

As I was accustomed to the constellation of modern amenities that keep us comfy, these conditions were almost comical by comparison. To wash my body, I had to take a big bucket to the middle of a courtyard and fill it with water to be carried back to my "shower", which was actually a cement room with a water spicket. But every time, without fail, I would splash so much water from my bucket it was nearly empty by the time I made it back to my room. What may seem like menial first world dissonance, felt then, like I was stepping into a daring adventure— armed with independence and eagerness. One day I was walking down the street and I saw a sign that said, "Ayurveda Clinic—appointments for foreigners." The term foreigner referred to me. It meant that the proprietors spoke English and welcomed tourists. I did not know anything about Ayurveda, I had never even heard of it. But the appointment was only thirty minutes and four dollars so I decided, what the hey, I have nothing to lose. I sat across from a big boned Indian woman who wore a sweater and jeans. She had enormous bug eyes, with one lazy eye that veered off away from where she was looking. She spoke "Hinglish", half English and half Hindi. She asked to see my tongue as she grabbed my hand to take my pulse. She asked me a few questions like: "Have you always been this thin?" and "Do you get hungry a lot?" I didn't know where she was going with the questions, but I appeased her inquiries. "No, I haven't always been very thin and no ma'am I don't get hungry a lot." Hunger used to be a bad concept in my world, so I terminated the thought. I wasn't about to admit to her that I had incessant gnawing hunger pangs. After scribbling down a few notes on a small piece of paper, she looked up at me and said I was Pitta/Vata. These words meant nothing to me. I had never heard them before. She proceeded to tell me that because of my strong fire element I can get very hungry and angry easily. I immediately turned beat red and shouted, "What?! No, I don't!" I heard myself and wanted to recoil. Oh my goodness, I just got very angry. Very easily. Hmmm, maybe this woman was on to something. She continued. She told me to avoid spicy foods, coffee, onions, tomatoes, and alcohol. I loved those things by the way. Then she told me to stay out of the heat, try not to be competitive, and never sunbathe because my skin is sensitive. *Woman! First you call me out on being hungry and prone to anger and now you're telling me to eliminate all my favorite foods and activities?! We are not off to a good start!* It was time to go. I brought my hands to prayer over my heart, bowed, grabbed the paper, stuffed it in my back pocket, and left. During that trip we visited an Ayurvedic clinic where the doctor was dignified and poised in his appearance. He invited us into his clean and air conditioned office. I know clean and air conditioned might not seem deserving of a mention, but believe me, after four weeks in 100 degree weather, covered in flies, this was heaven.

He proceeded to take our pulses and revealed to us things we already knew. The enthralling part was, how did he know these things? He knew I was prone to having bouts of constipation and anxiety. He knew I was ambitious, but got irritable and impatient easily. He knew coffee gave me heartburn. He knew all of this by taking my pulse! Needless to say, I was aroused. Maggie and I left feeling inspired by this system of medicine that was somehow covert or dismissed in our part of the world. Jump ahead several months. I'm at home in the town I grew up in—sleeping, one of those deep sleeps where the outer world disappears. Suddenly, I hear this voice as clear as day. The voice says, "Study Ayurveda. You must study Ayurveda." I open my eyes. It's just me. Me and pillows. Who said that? The voice sounded like a Guru or Gandhi or someone important. I'm not arguing with that guy. It was 3am. I jumped out of bed, got on the computer and immediately started researching Ayurveda schools. To my surprise, there were not many schools and they were all very expensive. I decided to go on Amazon and order every single Ayurveda book I could get my hands on. My mom was sweet enough to buy them for me as an early Christmas present. That Christmas morning was hilarious. I opened my gifts and every book had dog-eared pages, highlights, sticky notes and writing in the margins. My mom said, "Sweetpea, did you open your gifts early?" Oh I did. I dove into those books with a overwhelming curiosity for every word and meaning. There was no way I could wait until Christmas to read my gifts. Maybe this is what the bug-eyed lady meant when she said I was always hungry. Maybe that's what the poised doctor said when he hinted I was impatient. Whatever the case may be, I had fallen in love. I felt like I was downloading all the information I needed to help me understand myself and the other individuals in my life. I even began to see glimpse of how the universe functions. I know that may sound like a bold statement, but it's sincere. It didn't take long for everyone around me to catch wind of my new found interest. Initially, I held a free workshop at my yoga studio. Over fifty people attended. I was eager to share everything I recently uncovered. I talked for hours while facilitating Ayurvedic quizzes, giving suggestions, and answering questions. Much to my delight, my passion sparked a genuine interest for Ayurveda in my yoga community. I carried on with my yoga studies learning about philosophy, breathing, meditation, and how to contort my body into unusual shapes. My yoga program ended six weeks later, but I wasn't ready to go. I felt like I had just tasted an appetizer and I was still starving for more. I wanted to be further immersed in this culture and way of living. Fortunately, the yoga school invited me to stay free of charge and help teach the next course. I was elated. The only downfall was that I was out of books. I had read every fiction, non-fiction, poetry, philosophy, and romance novel on the shelf. There was only one book store in town and I had read almost all of the books they carried. The final remaining book was none other than a book about Ayurveda. I was less than enthused to read it, but I needed something to entertain me at night—after all there was no TV. After flipping through the pages, I found the principles to be interesting but relatively hard to understand. I didn't fully grasp it. I finished the book, gave it to a friend and never thought about it again. Well, until now.

Sixteen months later, I found myself back in America where I slowly molded my life into a career teaching yoga. I began leading dozens of classes a week at studios, gyms and corporate events. I was doing what I loved but was itching for another adventure. My time in India had left such a lasting impact on my life, I decided to go back. But this time, I went with my friend, Maggie, to Kerala, which is in southern India. Little did I know, Kerala is actually the motherland of Ayurveda. The streets are littered with signs for Ayurvedic herbs, massages, foods, and clinics. I wasn't particularly interested in Ayurveda, but you don't have to twist my arm to get a massage. Services in India are very affordable, so I indulged. I received all sorts of fascinating Ayurveda treatments. I had oil rubbed all over my body, dripped on my forehead, and administered into my nose and ears. I received treatments where my body was rubbed down in herbs and clay, patted with sacks of plants and spices. I even had tiny domes of warm melted butter (ghee) poured into my eyes. I am not kidding, I tried it all. And I loved it. I was not going to stop eating spicy food, drinking coffee or sunbathing, but this I could manage. A few months later, my friend Maggie received an email from a physician in our community who owns an Urgent Care Clinic. He was reaching out to see if my friend would teach yoga as part of a corporate wellness program, and added "P.S. Do you know anyone who is knowledgeable in Ayurveda?" My friend showed me the email and I immediately leaped up to respond to his request. Here's a tale of serendipity. The physician offered to pay for my formal Ayurveda education (remember, that's the same education I couldn't afford so opted for self study instead). In return, I would to bring Eastern Medicine into our community while working at his urgent care clinic to pay him back. Deal! I studied at Kripalu School of Ayurveda in Massachusetts. I opened my Ayurveda clinic under the Urgent Care Doctor's office. I can't help but think there are invisible forces in the universe that are powerful beyond measure. Forces that support us and guide us. Forces that clear paths, create intentional hurdles and invite us to fulfill a purpose we ourselves may only be on the cusp of recognizing. I spent the next several years expanding my business to my own clinic, studying intricate aspects of Ayurveda like pulse diagnosis, Marma (like acupuncture) and psychology. I traveled back to India to intern at an Ayurvedic Research Center. I created an organic

Ayurvedic product line for self-care called Wellblends, and I came full circle to teaching Ayurveda to yoga students who participate in very similar courses as the one I originally took in India years ago. Perhaps I wasn't initially attracted to Ayurveda because I wasn't ready for it. Maybe it wasn't delivered to me in a way that resonated with me. Maybe I didn't understand it. For whatever reason, it was not love at first sight. But now, Ayurveda is integral to my life as my heartbeat. These principles and tools have changed my life—not only because I got to make a career out of it and help people on a daily basis, but because Ayurveda gave me the framework and language I needed to understand my body, mind, and emotions. It guided me to realize the shifts and changes that come with everyday life, the turning of seasons, and the metamorphosis into new phases of life and how to adapt to these natural undulations of time.

You'll discover this book is split into two sections. Section ONE: Dosha Balancing Lifestyle is all about discovering your constitution, understanding the mind-body connection, and incorporating harmonious activities, such as self-care practices, and daily rituals into your life. This includes daily habits, meditation, breathing practices, yoga, intention setting, and cultivating awareness around how our thoughts impact our reality. Part TWO is Nutrition and Healing. In this section we'll debunk the false information we've been fed regarding food and diet. We'll uncover the key concepts of Ayurvedic nutrition, and learn how to eat for our Dosha. We'll address cravings, emotional eating, stress eating, and how food effects our psychology. This section includes meal plans, Dosha pacifying diets, recipes, and home remedies for common imbalances. This book is meant to be a compressive guide that will accompany you as you integrate Ayurveda into your beautiful life. I hope you enjoy reading the pages of this book as much as enjoyed writing them.

CHAPTER ONE

Meet Ayurveda

"The doctor of the future will give no medicine, but will interest his patients in the care of the human frame, in nutrition and in the cause and prevention of disease."

—Thomas Edison

"Did you know that your soul is composed of harmony?"

—Leonardo da Vinci

AYURVEDA REMINDS YOU of what you instinctually know to be true. I clearly remember my first day at Kripalu School of Ayurveda. I arrived with all my textbooks, notebooks, binders, and thirty pens in every imaginable color. I was so eager to learn. I enthusiastically snaked my way through the rows of chairs to find my perfect seat among a crowded room of peers. I sat down, twiddled my fingers and stared at the platform at the front of the room. The dean of the school approached the podium to welcome us. Her greeting was warm and allowed my anxious, clammy palms to dry up. As she prepared us for the journey ahead, she said, "Everything you are about to learn... you already know." What?!?! My inner monologue yelled, "Huh? I rearranged my work, finances, and my life to be here and you are telling me I already know everything I'm going to learn? Then what the heck am I doing here?" I took a deep breath. The spikes in my gut softened back into their usual smooth form and I relaxed. As the year progressed, I learned the ins, outs, whys, and hows of Ayurveda, but the dean was absolutely correct. The textures of Ayurveda felt familiar from the beginning. With each concept I grasped, I connected new dots and things began to click. This click tends to happen when we make sense of what we already know. Ayurveda is intuitive. The fabric of the science is woven from fundamental laws and truths of nature. Ayurveda allows us to truly feel the textures, understand nuances and learn how to skillfully thread invaluable components of our lives together. We develop strategies to live healthier lives. In teaching and working with clients, I have the privilege of watching people integrate Ayurveda into their lives on daily basis. I see them light up as they connect the dots and awaken to their renewed understanding. The most common phrase I hear through their refreshed smiles is, "It just makes sense." I'm going to hold your hand as we jump into this big pool of the nitty-gritty, the ABCs of Ayurveda. It is important to wrap our heads around the fundamentals before diving into the nuances of the science and lifestyle. Even the masterful poet, Rumi had to learn the alphabet. It is because of his soulful interpretation of the building blocks of language that we still ride the inspiring reverberations of his poetry. We will equip ourselves with the ABCs of Ayurveda so that our life and wellness feel like living poetry.

What is Ayurveda? Ayurveda is pronounced "R-U-Veda." Ayurveda is a Sanskrit word that means, the science of life or wisdom of longevity. Sanskrit is the language of Ancient India. Along with Hebrew, it is one of the oldest languages. This natural and traditional medicine of India originated about 5,000 years ago. Chinese and Tibetan medicines both trace their roots back to Ayurveda. The original knowledge was realized by Rishis or seers. Rishis, or seers are essentially enlightened people who received and understood remarkable amounts of information and wisdom that was channeled to them by the whispers of the universe. In a way, they are like spiritual geniuses. Later, the knowledge was compiled into texts called the Charaka Samhita, which is basically the holy grail of Eastern Medicine. Additional classical texts include Sushruta Samhita and Ashtanga Hridya. The scope of Ayurveda is broad, rich, and thorough. Traditionally, there are eight branches of Ayurveda: internal medicine, surgery, E.N.T., pediatrics & gynecology, psychiatry, toxicology, rejuvenation, immunity & anti-aging, and aphrodisiacs & fertility. Ayurveda is truly holistic in that it addresses the entire spectrum of the human experience on the physical, mental, energetic, and spiritual levels. Like Yoga, while Ayurveda is ancient, it is by no means esoteric. The ideals and applications of Ayurveda are fully functional in today's modern world.

The first aim in Ayurveda medicine is to protect the health of a healthy person. Ayurveda will help you grasp complete wellness through diet, lifestyle and the achievement of balance. These dimensions spill over into your relationships, career and overall happiness. With this 360 degree comprehensive approach, you will be able to care for the common imbalances that we all experience from time to time. Along the way, you will learn to optimize your strengths and sidestep new ailments before they fully manifest. If you are currently in the midst of a serious illness, allow this book to serve as a support mechanism. The information in this book is here to heighten your awareness and broaden your skill set for bringing wellness into your life. This book is not intended to cure disease. Notify your physician of any changes you choose to implement regarding your nutrition and lifestyle. Regardless of where you fall on the spectrum of harmony or disharmony, resist the urge to make radical changes. No one achieves balance by being extreme. Let the information wash over you. Trust that whatever feels right and saturates into the way you live is correct. We all learn and adjust at our own tempo. Honor your intuition and personal time table. If this book piques your interest, return to these pages often. Allow this book to serve as your consistent wellness companion. Similar to yoga, the practice of Ayurveda will constantly morph, fade, return, and deepen. Should you fall in love with Ayurveda, I encourage you to go seek more.

Read more books, visit a practitioner for a personal consultation, slather yourself in turmeric and drink chai tea. The paths are endless. The journey is meant to be enjoyed.

> *"Find a place inside where there's joy, and the joy will burn out the pain."*
>
> **—Joseph Campbell**

Health Care or Disease Management? There is a time and place for Western medicine and intricate protocols. If God forbid

I get into an accident, please do not rub herbs on me and tell me to go to bed on time. Take me to the hospital. Physicians do amazing things. They save lives. Modern medicine has achieved fantastic triumphs. However, I do believe our culture has a tendency to lunge for synthetic drugs more than necessary. We seek health, happiness, repair, and fulfillment in the form of little white capsules. The overuse of pharmaceutical drugs has become a perilous epidemic. I think a more accurate title for our modern health care system would be, disease management. In our present system, most people go to the doctor when they are already sick or injured. In chronic and acute cases, modern medicine has the capacity to alleviate pain and mitigate premature death, However, research validates that poor nutrition and chronic stress are responsible for the majority of modern illnesses. Knowing this, our approach to health should be on prevention. We do not have wait until there is a crisis to take action.

Nourishing ourselves mind, body, and spirit with intention, and by practicing a more mindful approach to self-care will protect and recapture our birthright. It is our birthright to be well. I am sure yoga has served as a place of solace, a retreat from the daily demands of modern life for you. Yoga's sister science, Ayurveda will serve as an additional resource for you to create the life of peace and health you desire and deserve. I am reminded of a story I heard in a lecture by mind-body physician, Dr.Deepak Chopra. He described a study where dozens of flies where put into a container. After some time, the lid was taken off of the container. In reality, the flies were free to exit the container and fly away without limitations. But do you know what happened? The flies stayed. They remained in their crowded, confined space because they conceded to an agreement that the container was their reality. Over the course of the study, only one fly acted as a pioneer who flew away to explore new spaces and amplified levels of freedom and awareness. We do not have to stay in the container of a cultural agreement that lends itself to stressful lives, sickness, and intoxicants or the use of synthetic drugs to perhaps feel better and god-willing, relax. We do not have to tolerate an intolerable lifestyle. We are not prisoners.

We are pioneers. We are like the lone courageous fly. We have the capacity to remove the lid from the glass ceiling. We can draft a new agreement where health, and contentment are not just for the lucky or blessed. Health and contentment are intrinsic in our purpose for being here. Right here. Right now. We are signing a new agreement that declares health and contentment are our birthrights.

> *"To make happy is to heal."*
>
> **—The Course in Miracles**

We are the creators of a new paradigm. To paraphrase Abraham, from *The Law of Attraction:* we focus on the body, not because the body is the most important aspect of our being, but because we and everyone we know has one. A body, whether in good health or poor can be changed. Any physical state can always be augmented to match the state that is desired by the individual. This principle demonstrates that we should focus on the state we prefer. The law of attraction illustrates that we are magnets and we draw to us that which we most dominantly think about. Out thoughts constantly strengthen our magnet. To get what you prefer, the law states you must place our attention on the preferable. If you want to be prosperous, you must focus on prosperity. Someone who constantly thinks about scarcity will not attract abundance. Whereas someone who thinks about abundance will charge the magnet that brings prosperity into their reality. Someone who wishes to be thin will not become thin by thinking they are fat. Wayne Dyer says, "You will see it when you believe it." We can launch change by being deliberate with the thoughts and language that support our beliefs. I love the quote, "Be careful what you say to yourself. You are listening." The body is obedient. The body will appease what you constantly request. Hold yourself accountable for your thoughts.

Reiterate what you want. Do not get me wrong, this is not all about positive thinking, hocus-pocus, or rainbow narrative. Our thoughts have to be actionable. Sitting around and thinking about money will not make you rich any faster than sitting around thinking about water will quench your thirst. But how can we know where to place our efforts and actions if we do not first become definite as to what it is we want? And as importantly, absolute about we believe we deserve?

Throughout the pages of this book I will season the chapters with, "I AM" statements. These statements are not expectations or goals. We use this vibrationally charge descriptive language to help solidify what it is that we are attracting into our lives. The, "I AM" affirmation serves as a potent power source for you to charge up whatever it is you wish to manifest in your life. Ralph Waldo Emerson said, "The ancestor to every action is a thought." I AM statements help us to internalize our deepest desires.

PAUSE FOR AFFIRMATION

"I am open to learning, loving and healing."

Prioritizing and respecting the value of what you eat and how you live will open you up to an inner pharmacy. The bedrock of these Ayurvedic principles rest in making positive choices in regards to the food you consume, and the lifestyle you choose to entertain. Nutrition and lifestyle are integral to our wellbeing. We are enmeshed in the things we consume. What you choose to eat, think, say, do, and believe has the capacity to either narrow or broaden the distance between you and your highest self. You know you are in contact with your higher self when you feel your best. Health happens on a moment to moment basis. The opportunity to feel your best is baked into the cake of the very thought you are having right now. And now. And now. Every moment is impressionable.

Ayurvedic medicine addresses and corrects the sick, but is health centric. Health centric implies that using these principles will enhance the existing state of ones wellbeing. With Ayurveda you can lift your current reference point for what you consider to be healthy, you can raise the baseline for your personal degree of wellbeing. When I began this journey, I considered myself healthy. Sure I had my occasional complaint such as a painful or missed period, foggy brain, blemished skin, a poor night's sleep, or absent bowel movement, but I did not have any diagnosed diseases. Prior to Ayurveda, if I would have filled out a survey asking me if I thought I was healthy I would have ticked the, "yes" box without hesitation. It was not until I began to apply the principles of Ayurveda that I fine-tuned my health in such a way that the bar for personal wellbeing elevated to new heights. I remember thinking, "Oh this is what healthy feels like".

Have you ever been to the doctor because you felt lethargic, heavy, or just, "off" only to discover that your blood tests or scans revealed nothing was wrong? Intuitively you know something was out of whack, but because it couldn't be diagnosed you were left without solutions. This can be incredibly frustrating. According to Ayurveda there are six stages of disease. Stages one through three translates into vague signs with growing discomfort or intensity. For example, feeling tired, turns into a dull headache, then progresses to a piercing migraine. The current Western model does not address the disease until it has reached the fourth or fifth stage. By this stage the imbalance has exacerbated to a full blown disease, it has reached its completely identifiable form. This is the stage where modern medicine can diagnose the disease with a label and attempt a treatment method according to standard protocols and pharmaceutical drugs. Ayurveda focuses on catching the disease before it reaches full manifestation. Ayurveda doesn't treat the disease. The approach is personal. Ayurveda treats the person.

> *"The first question an Ayurvedic physicians asks is not, 'What disease does my patient have?' but 'Who is my patient?' By 'who' the physician does not mean your name, but how are you constituted."*
>
> **—Deepak Chopra M.D.**

Ayurveda teaches us to recognize disharmony before reaching the latter stages of pathology, because once a disease if full blown it is more difficult to treat. The body's self repair mechanisms will struggle to reverse the disharmony without the support of drugs or surgery. These more dramatic interventions are often accompanied by complicated side effects. If we are not educated and equipped on how to spot an imbalance and target ailments early on, we will likely resort the familiar options we find in doctor"s offices, hospitals and little orange bottles. Learning how to identify an imbalance can save us from necessary treatment options.

For example, I used to get excruciatingly painful periods. I would curl into a ball of agony, take a menstrual pain relievers, or try to ignore it and plough through my pain. I masked and ignored my body's signal for so long that my period gave up on me and stopped coming. I went to a gynecologist who diagnosed my condition as amenorrhea. She tried to prescribe me birth control pills and synthetic hormones to kick start my cycle. At that point I was well into my holistic studies, so I did not resonate with that form of treatment. I ended up taking an Ayurvedic approach to reviving my menstrual cycle, and nourishing my reproductive system. But, because I did not recognize my symptoms as a request to find balance earlier on, the treatment was more time and labor intensive than I would have preferred. In order to revive my cycle, I had to do daily oil enemas, drink herbal wines, swallow herbs, modify my diet, learn to rest, and drink four to six cups of herbal tea a day. My cycle returned to normal and came without pain after about five months of following the ayurveda treatment plan, but I could have regulated and nourished my reproductive system earlier, and with fewer steps had I acknowledged and understood the signs of imbalance sooner. The secret is listening closely in the early stages. That kind of listening will allow us to dodge needless suffering.

"Health is much more dependent on our habits and nutrition than on medicine."

—John Lubbock

How Does It Work? Ayurveda grabs ahold of two fundamental factors of daily life: food and rhythm. We all eat (food), and as the sunrises and the sunsets we all function in accordance to some sort of schedule (or rhythm). Striking a balance with our nutritional habits and our daily rhythms are key factors to health. We are all uniquely entangled in intimate relationships with these two variables. Ayurveda intelligently adapts these core components of daily life in a way that works to our advantage. We can use the tools Ayurveda offers us to design wellness by crafting a balanced approach to daily food choices and daily rhythms.

Ayurveda does not need to be practiced exclusively. Ayurveda is a medical system in itself, however it could also be used to complement other medical approaches. For example, a type 2 diabetic could take insulin, but also use cinnamon to regulate glucose (sugar) levels. Someone suffering from arthritis could take their anti-inflammatory medications if they want to, but by adding Golden Milk (primarily turmeric and ginger) they will likely drop the need to refill their prescription. I often see people who have struggled with insomnia for years and by adopting a nightly routine of oil massage, chamomile tea, or Golden Milk—they find relief. People who battle anxiety find support and ease through establishing stable routines and breathing exercises. Acne can be cleared with a natural paste of herbs like turmeric and an herb called neem (ingredients in Radiant Me Complexion Mask). The pages of this book are filled with ways to use everything from what's on the end of your fork, to what's on the soles of your feet as medicine.

> *"Without right food and lifestyle, medicine is of no use. With right food and lifestyle, medicine is of no need."*
>
> **—Charaka Samhita**

The key here is to create an atmosphere that supports healing. We want to adapt our daily acts and habits to function as complimentary patterns to promote healing. For example, if you are taking decongestants, but eating mucus forming foods like Alfredo for dinner and frozen yogurt for dessert (both items are intensely mucus forming), even in taking the strongest medicines available, you are breaking even at best because as the medications reduce the congestion, the wrong foods breed more of it. Someone suffering with depression may take an antidepressant, but if they are eating lifeless food and dragging their feet to a job they hate, then they are missing the peripheral support that could lift them out of their state of lassitude. If someone struggles with constipation, taking laxatives can provide acute relief whereas understanding the qualities of food, eating for ones constitution, starting the day with warm water, and taking aloe vera gel at night would promote regular eliminations without habit forming stimulants. Think of medicine as a seed, and your food and lifestyle as soil. If one's food and lifestyle are in incongruent with balance, than the soil is denatured or toxic. No seed, regardless strength, can thrive in soil that is denatured or toxic. We must take care of our soil instead of always reaching for another seed.

Like Yoga, Ayurveda has Stood the Test of Time for a Reason. In an ever quickening world that is crowded with chemicals, pollutants and stressors there is no better time to draw upon these profound truths for guidance, inspiration and perspective. Epigenetic's states that we are the sum of our experiences. Allow your life to be your medicine. best state, your health, and your happiness are at your fingertips. Whether you adopt Ayurveda as a complete system for medical healing, preventative care, template for how to live your life, consort to your yoga practice, or as a method to slow the natural process of wear and tear that occurs with aging —Ayurveda will earn it's place in your life as a valuable friend, resource, and guidepost for insight and health.

> *"When you have a high degree of integration you don't have to make uncomfortable choices. Your mind, heart and body act in harmony and cooperate to fulfill your desires. Everything you think, feel and do ultimately has to connect. Otherwise, you feel scattered and unstable. This little understood but key component of healthiness cannot be put into a small white pill."*
>
> **—Maharishi Ayurveda**

Doshas, Elements and the Mind-Body Constitutions: Do not let these cute, unfamiliar words throw you off. As you read and stumble upon new words, just note that they are Sanskrit words. Much like we use Latin in the modern medicine world, we use Sanskrit in the world of Ayurveda. Every unfamiliar word will be clearly defined for you. The language of Sanskrit reads like a poem, each word holds great meaning and substance—therefore I might use several English words to define one Sanskrit word. The meaning behind these terms will seamlessly integrate into your field of understanding. Let's look at the Doshas. Physical, mental and emotional characteristics come together to reveal your unique mind-body constitution. The constitutions are referred to as Doshas. The word Dosha means, that which can be vitiated, or that which can be impaired. We all have a personalized Doshic makeup, therefor, it is in our inherent design to experience continuous states of fluctuation, transition and evolution. Doshas are combinations of elements. The elements are ether, air, fire, water and earth. Ether is space, such as the space in our stomachs when we are hungry, the space in our joints that lend us extended mobility, or the space between thoughts when we finally get a chance to relax. Air presents itself ubiquitously…when we breathe, pass gas, or move quickly like the wind. Fire appears in the body as heat—like the hot/acidic atmosphere of our internal digestive organs, (hydrochloric acids and enzymes are hot), or the warm feeling of an inflamed joint. The water quality surfaces as tears, sweat, and urine to name a few. Last, but not least, earth translates into our structure. Our strong muscles and insulating adipose tissue. Every element makes a specific contribution. All of the elements work together and serve the united purpose, of supporting the whole of you.

We all have all five elements in us, but the proportions of each element provide us with our Doshic makeup. And guess whatour Doshas shift. There is nothing aberrant about derailing from time to time. If Dosha means, that which can be impaired, it is in our design to have impaired balance from time to time. We are perfectly imperfect. The benefit of understanding the Doshas, or the mind-body constitutions is that you will have a better idea of how, and when you have a likelihood to go out of balance. Equipped with this new found awareness, you will be able to spot the imbalance earlier, and correct it gracefully. Understanding the Doshas is a lot like understanding a compass. With a compass, you can chart your direction from a clearer vantage point.

You my friend, are a personalized blend of Vata, Pitta and Kapha. Your unique blend is referred to as your Doshic makeup or constitution. Imbalances in the body and mind surface when the Doshas are out of balance. An imbalance in your Doshas can present in a number of ways. One Dosha may become too prevalent, or one may be neglected and lose the strength it needs to support you. Cultivating a life of balance will keep our Doshas balanced. One of my favorite teachers and authors, Claudia Welch wrote the book, *Balance your hormones, Balance your life.* When she came to speak at Kripalu, she revealed to us that she actually wanted to title her book, "Balance your life, Balance your hormones", because more often than not, imbalanced hormones are not the cause of a chaotic life. A chaotic life is the cause of imbalanced hormones. The same is true for the Doshas. When life is imbalanced, the Doshas are out of balance—the elemental quantities become disproportionate to ones inherent constitution (meaning the way your body-mind blue print intends for you to be.) For example, I am 50% Vata and 50% Pitta (with only a smidgen of Kapha). If I do neglect to take good care of myself by becoming too busy, eating too many raw foods, and doing too many activities my Vata may sky rocket to 60 or 80%. This would lend itself to a host of Vata imbalances (such as the painful, absent and irregular periods I mentioned earlier). Or perhaps a friend is 80% Pitta, 5% Kapha and 5% Vata, she would have to be mindful of her food and lifestyle choices to maintain balance. Her high Pitta will drive her to overwork, compete with herself and others, fuel up on things she craves like spicy foods, coffee and alcohol. Her predominately Pitta constitution left to it's own devices will rise beyond measure. An imbalance in Pitta could cause her to wrestle with heat related issues such as irritability, impatience, and ulcers to name a few.

The goal is not to achieve equal parts Vata, Pitta and Kapha. The goal is not to achieve anything really. The goal is to understand yourself. Understanding your unique constitution and living in a way that compliments your constitution will give you insight to better position yourself to recapture, maintain and fully enjoy your wellbeing.

"The more in harmony you are with the flow of your own existence, the more magical life becomes."

—Adyashanti

Return to Your True Nature:

Returning to your True Nature will allow you to live in concord with the universal code that best supports you. Your mind and body offer pathological wisdom. You are privy to this information. You were born with a genetic blueprint or mind-body layout that is exclusive to you. This is called your "Prakriti", or True Nature. Your True Nature is essential a printout of your constitutional—Doshic makeup . Several factors came into play during the creation of your specific True Nature. Your parents constitution, the time of year you were born, the time of year you were conceived, and your Karma (effects from past actions) all played a role in the formation of your True Nature.

The first seven years of your life were formative because ones childhood is instrumental in the development of ones physicality and behavioral traits. Everything that happened during those initial seven years of life created an impression, much like bare feet on wet cement. Around year seven, the cement dried and your True Nature was solidified. Depending on your age, there is certainly distance between how you were at seven years of age, and how you are today. Over that course of time—life happened. Environmental factors, food and lifestyle choices, unexpected events, stressors, sorrows, joy, and all things that keep life interesting transpired. All of these occurrences lead you to where you are now. Now you are at your Current State or "Virkriti". If the events of your life were largely in alignment with your True Nature, meaning you made great food and lifestyle choices, your stress was minimal, and your environment was supportive — chances are, you feel pretty good. Essentially, your Doshic makeup is balanced. But, if life deviated off course, meaning your food and lifestyle choices were not the greatest, stress was booming, you had an accident, your environment was harsh and the like, then you have deviated from your True Nature. Deviating from your True Nature can cause physical and mental disharmonies, and disease. The closer you get to your True Nature, the better you feel.

> *"According to Ayurvedic principles, by understanding oneself, by identifying one's own constitution, and by recognizing sources of Doshic aggravation, one can not only follow proper guidelines to cleanse, purify and prevent disease, but also uplift oneself into a realm of awareness previously unknown.*
>
> **—Vasant Lad**

Doshas: Our First Glance at the Mind-Body Constitutions…

Vata: Vata is comprised of ether and air. Sometimes referred to as Wind. The meaning of Vata is, "That which moves." Movement is the driving force of life. Our breath, heartbeat, and circulation all give thanks to movement. Speech, mobility and the transference of thoughts all happen because of movement. Movement is a key ingredient to life. In fact, there was a study where a group of scientist came together to create a ecosphere. As an experiment, they created a contained environment with proper amounts of soil, water and fire. They made sure the air was fresh, and all the carefully selected plants and animals had everything they needed to thrive. The temperatures were correct, suitable food sources were accessible—everything was is place. All of the scientist went home and when they came back in the morning they were astounded to find that many of the plants died and the animals were sick. They scientist grabbed their heads in confusion. They had dotted all the I's and crossed all the T's. What went wrong? They forgot wind. They forgot the breeze. Devoid of wind that governs circulation and movement of air, everything died. As you can see Vata is vital to the presence of life on earth.

Physically Vata people have small bones, dry hair and skin, smaller or darker eyes, and inconsistencies, for example their face might not be fully symmetrical. Vata types can be extreme, so either very tall or very short—they may have very curly hair or extremely straight hair. Their minds are creative and adaptable. In balance, people with a lot of Vata in their constitution are inventive, easily excitable and movement oriented. They know how to temper their energy as to not exert all their energy at once. They are aware that crowded schedules and minimal structure wreck havoc on their energy and health. Out of balance, Vata types have a tendency to have dry and crackly joints (crepitus). They become constipated, bloated and gassy easily. Their minds become hyperactive, unfocused and forgetful. A disharmonious Vata may experience anxiety, restless sleep and insomnia. You may be Vata if you often find yourself ruining late and feeling like life is frenzy. Each constitution comes with its own terms of hunger and digestion. Vata digestion is irregular. People with Vata digestion may be famished one day and forget to eat the next day. Vata governs movement, such as circulation, breath, speech and mobility, so Vata types like activity whether it be mental, oral or physical. But excess stimulation can tax a Vata types nervous system, leading to anxiety or exhaustion. We want to keep Vata in balance, because as Vata is wind—a breeze is refreshing, whereas an over abundance of wind, such as a tornado is calamitous.

Pitta: Pitta is comprised of fire and water. The meaning of Pitta is, "That which transforms." As the driver of transformation, Pitta has a strong metabolism for food and thoughts. Pittas are sharp. They are sharp in the bellies, i.e.: hungry for food, and sharp in their minds, i.e.: hungry for knowledge. People with a strong dose of Pitta are generally medium build and develop muscle tone easily. They may have fine, light or red hair. They may experience premature graying or balding because the fire rises to their minds, and burns their hair follicles. Their skin may be sensitive, slightly red, freckled or blemished. Pittas usually have green or sharp eyes (when a Pitta is looking at you, you know it). Pitta's potent aptitude for transformation and metabolism provides them with a strong capacity to digest and assimilate nutrients and information. Mentally, someone with a strong Pitta constitution is bright, ambitious, and charismatic. A balanced Pitta will tend to be goal oriented and successful. A balanced Pitta knows that they must take care to not over work, because their natural drive can drive them straight towards a short fuse, and a feeling of burn out. Out of balance Pittas may experience inflammation. Any kind of 'itis' in the body, skin irritations, light sensitivity, heartburn, acid indigestion and loose stools. Psychologically, an overheated Pitta may become competitive, judgmental and over zealous about work pursuits. A person with a predominantly Pitta constitution will have a hearty appetite and efficient metabolism. You may be a Pitta if people refer to you as a "Go Getter".

Kapha: Kapha is comprised of earth and water. The meaning of Kapha is, "That which holds." Because Kapha is formed from the two heaviest elements, earth and water, Kapha has a density. This density gives us structure and stability. Kapha holds all the moving parts in place. Kapha provides protection. Kapha types are loyal and patient. They're typically stable and reliable. Their bodies are full, sturdy, thick and strong. They have big bright eyes, fuller hair, larger lips, breasts and buttocks, and denser bones. Their digestion is slower, so Kapha types need to be cautious in the areas of weight related issues, as well as respiratory issues like allergies and asthma. Because Kapha is heavy, too much Kapha can lead to heavy behaviors and feelings such as: laziness, complacency and even depression. In balance, Kapha types make loyal employees and sweet homemakers. You may be Kapha if people refer to you as, "Someone they can rely on."

Dreams, Spending Habits, and Careers…Each Dosha will express its qualities in all facets of life. This includes the way we dream, spend money, and earn a living. Vatas tend to have action packed dreams. They are often flying, traveling, or racing around. Pittas tend to have lifelike dreams. They are troubleshooting problems or pragmatically moving through an adventure scene. Kaphas tend to not remember their dreams, or they have romantic or sensual dreams involving water and romance. Vatas are quick to spend money. They'll make spontaneous, spitfire purchases frequently. Pittas tend to invest in luxury items, practical items, or something that will evolve their position—such as furthering their education. Kapha's tend to hold onto their money. They're the best savers. In regards to career; Vatas enjoy creative gigs. They gravitate towards being teachers, dancers, writers, musicians, and designers. Pittas like positions of power and prestige, such as being a leadership, an entrepreneur, a doctor, lawyer, professor, or politician. Kaphas do well in supporting roles. They like to assist and take care of others. They make great executive assistance, chefs, nurses, caretakers, and hospitality workers.

Celebrities…Reveal Doshas!

Vatas: Kelly Ripa, Gwyneth Paltrow, Haley Barry, Audrey Hepburn, and Taylor Swift.

Pittas: Nicole Kidman, Cameron Diaz, Reese Witherspoon, Sandra Bullock, Princess Diana, Hillary Clinton, and Michelle Obama.

Kaphas: Oprah, Beyonce, Marilyn Monroe, Rachel Ray, Scarlet Johansen, and Maya Angelou.

CHAPTER TWO

Discover Doshas

"When the mind and body are in harmony, the mind works better and gives the body physical prowess."

—Caroline Prohosky

DISCOVERING MY DOSHA: Here is a simple questionnaire to help you determine your mind-body constitution. There are two ways to complete the quiz. First, answer the quiz in accordance to how you were as a child, and throughout the earlier portion of your life. This will give you an idea about your 'Prakriti', or True Nature. This will indicate your tendencies and characteristics when you are in your purest state, the state when you feel your best and, "like yourself." Then, answer the questions in accordance to how you're feeling now (recent six months.) Answering the quiz according to your present conditions will give you a basic idea of your 'Vrikriti', or Current State. For some of you, your Current State may be largely similar to your True Nature. If this is the case, you likely feel pretty good. You may have the occasional ache or pain, digestive complaint, or slight weight fluctuation, but more or less—you are generally healthy. Doshic states are malleable, so they will not always remain in that desirable sweet spot that matches your True Nature. If your Current State indicates that your Doshic makeup has deviated from your True Nature, you're most likely experiencing noticeable imbalances. Your quiz will help you verify if your Current State is in concord with your True Nature, or not. Have no fears. Yes, there are a host of ways to fall out of balance, but luckily for us, there are just as many ways to return to balance. As you go through this questionnaire try not to over think your answers. There are questions where more than one answer can apply. Circle both. Even the way you move through this questionnaire will speak to your Dosha. Vata types have a tendency to want to move quickly, but have a hard time making a decision. Vata types may become overwhelmed. Don't let this happen. Just choose the option that feels best and move on. Pitta types will read and answer the questions methodically and precisely. Kapha types will take their time, enjoying the process and maybe even call a friend or family member to share the experience, and ask for guidance. There are no wrong answers. Make sure your answers are reflective of your reality, and not the way you want them to be. This is a great starting point. Have fun with it!

1. Physique

V) I am a slender person and I hardly gain weight. When I do gain weight it still obvious that I have a slight frame.
P) I am medium build. I develop muscle tone easily.
K) I am well built, and I gain weight no matter what I do.

2. Skin

V) My skin is dry and thin. I am prone
to itchy and wrinkly skin.
P) My skin looks flushed; I have lots of moles and freckles
on my body. I am prone to sunburns or acne.
K) My skin is smooth and soft, it has a tendency to be pale.
People say I am blessed with youthful looking skin.

3. Hair

V) My hair is dry, thin and brittle. It can look
frizzy or crispy if I don't tame it.
P) My hair may have a reddish hue, is fine or light in
color. It is not dry. I started get gray hair early in life.
K) My hair is thick, full, lustrous, and slightly
oily. I have voluminous hair.

4. Face

V) My face is oval, thin or bony. My features
are slightly asymmetrical.
P) My face is triangular (pointed chin,
prominent jaw line) or heart shaped.
K) My face is round or plump. I have large features.

5. Eyes

V) My eyes are small; they feel dry often and tend
to move quickly (looking around a lot).
P) My eyes are medium in shape. They may be blue
or green. People say I have a penetrating gaze.
K) My eyes are big and round in shape. I have full
eyelashes. People say I have warm and sweet eyes.

6. **Hands**

    V) My hands are generally dry and rough. I have slender fingers and dry and brittle nails.
    P) My hands are generally moist and pink. I have medium fingers and soft nails.
    K) My hands are generally firm and thick. I have thick fingers and strong & smooth nails.

7. **Joints and Bones**

    V) My joints are small, prominent bones, and often crack. My joints can feel dry and ache often. I have small bones.
    P) My joints are medium and loose. My joints can feel inflamed. I have medium sized bones.
    K) My joints are large, sturdy and have lots of muscle or tissue surrounding them. I can get joint pain because my extra weight adds pressure to them. I have large and sturdy bones.

8. **Activities**

    V) I am a very active person (always on the go—mind constantly thinking). I need a lot of movement in my day to feel comfortable.
    P) I like to think before I do anything. I tend to be competitive. I need to be good at the activities I choose.
    K) I am steady and graceful (I don't like to rush). I don't need excess movement in my day. I'm happy to take it easy.

9. Actions

V) I walk fast and talk fast. I'm usually in a hurry or I lose track of time.
P) My actions are very thoughtful and precise. I'm known for my punctuality.
K) I like a slower pace and I take my time to accomplish things. I'm usually not concerned with time, I'll get there.

10. Sleep

V) I rarely sleep soundly. I tend to toss and turn. I wake up early in the morning.
P) I am a light sleeper but if something wakes me up, I can go back to sleep easily. I wake up because I know I have things to accomplish.
K) I am a heavy sleeper. I love sleeping in.

11. Appetite

V) Varies, sometimes I feel hungry, sometimes not, I feel anxious if I don't eat.
P) I always feel hungry. If I don't eat I get irritable and angry.
K) I don't feel hunger pangs, but I love food. I can go without food easily for a day but I enjoy eating so I rarely miss a meal.

12. Bowel Movements

V) I tend to have constipation and can go a day or two without a bowel movement. I experience gas and bloating.

P) I am regular and sometimes stools are loose (tend to get diarrhea). I have experienced heartburn or acid indigestion.
K) I have no problem. I wake up to go to the bathroom, usually just once a day. Sometimes I feel heaviness after eating (especially if I eat too much).

13. Voice

V) My voice tends to be weak or hoarse. My voice tends to be high pitched.
P) I have a strong voice, I may get loud sometimes. My voice is direct.
K) My voice is deep, has good tone. My voice has a melodious quality. People tell me I sing well.

14. Emotions

V) I am a born worrier, I often feel anxious and nervous.
P) If things don't happen my way, I feel irritable and angry.
K) I am a happy person, very caring and loving.

15. Weather Preference

V) I love warm and humid weather. I dislike windy days.
P) I enjoy cool weather. I either really love or really despise hot weather.
K) I like warm but dry weather. Cool and cloudy days make me want to cuddle inside.

16. Career

V) I thrive when my work is creative,
fast paced and flexible.I would prefer
not to have a desk job.
P) I excel when I have a lot to manage and
achieve. I prefer a leadership role.
K) I enjoy caring for and helping other people.
I'm okay with a desk job, or supportive role.

17. Learning Style

V) I learn quickly, but forget quickly.
P) I grasp new ideas and concepts easily.
K) It takes me a while to absorb new
information, but I never forget it.

18. Actions

V) I tend to be spontaneous.
P) I am a list maker. I like to plan and organize.
K) I don't like to plan. I prefer to follow others.

19. Stamina

V) I like to do things in spurts. I have a
ton of energy then I get tired very easily.
My energy peaks and valleys.
P) I have medium stamina. I can accomplish
anything if I think it's important (despite
my energy or lack thereof)
K) I can work long hours and have endurance,
but sometimes I suffer from lassitude.

20. Mind

V) My mind gets restless easily. It can race in many directions at once.
P) I appreciate efficiency. I can get impatient easily.
K) It takes a lot to make me mad. I usually feel very calm.

21. Decision Making

V) I change my mind more often and will take time to make a decision.
P) I can make a decision easily. I am steadfast in my decisions.
K) I want others to make the decisions.

22. Personality

V) "Can I change my mind"?
P) "It's my way or the highway"
K) "Don't worry be happy"

23. Movement

V) I like action. I enjoy lots of movement.
P) I like to win. I like sportsmanship and competition.
K) I like to have fun. I take a chilled-out approach to persuits.

24. Health Problems

V) My symptoms are mainly pain, constipation, anxiety and depression.
P) I often get skin infections, fevers, heartburn, hypertension.
K) I tend to experience allergies, congestion, weight gain, and digestive problems.

25. Hobbies

V) I like art (drawing, painting, dance) and travel.
P) I like sports, politics, and things that
get my adrenaline pumping.
K) I like nature, gardening, reading, and cooking.

Tally: Go ahead and tally up your findings. Remember to do the quiz twice. Once for how you've been most of your life, particularly as a child (indicative of your True Nature). Then again as how you've been recently, in the past year or so (indicative of your Current State). This will give you a baseline understanding of your True Nature and Current State. It may be amusing to also have a close friend, family member or spouse take the quiz on your behalf as some of our answers can be subjective.

To be fair, when I first began studying and practicing Ayurveda my constitution was not absolute. I would gather slightly different findings based on the set of questions or clinician I visited. My findings were always in a similar ball park but nothing was set in stone. By focusing on aligning the Dosha that was creating the most pressing imbalance my constitution started to become more defined. It is not necessary to know your quote unquote exact constitution. What is important is becoming increasingly aware of the presence of each Dosha and how the Doshas are effecting you.

"There is no greater ecstasy than to know who you are."

—Osho

Let's get to know the nuances of the Doshas. Each Dosha has an affinity to a particular set of qualities we call Gunas. These qualities express themselves physically, mentally and emotionally. We utilize qualities to quantify and understand the origins and solutions for restoring and engaging balance.

VATA	PITTA	KAPHA
light	light	heavy
dry	oily	sticky
cold	hot	cold
rough	spreading	soft
irregular	pungent (spicy)	steady
quick	sharp	slow
changeable	acidic	dull

The qualities present themselves in a host of ways. We use the qualities to identify the Doshas and imbalances, as well as to treat the imbalances. For example, my friend Carrie visited me and expressed a concern for her thinning hair, forgetfulness, and trouble staying asleep at night. At first glance these symptoms might seem unrelated, but from the vantage point of Ayurveda, her concerns are categorized by the qualities of Vata. Her thinning hair was a result of rough and dry conditions. Her forgetfulness fell under the qualities of quick and changeable, and her trouble staying asleep were linked to the qualities of light and irregular.

When it comes to the qualities ... We Use Opposites to Create Balance. In Carrie's case, we needed to balance the presence of light, dry, cold, rough, irregular, quick and changeable qualities with their opposites: heavy, moisturized, warm, smooth, stable, and slow qualities. As life can be our medicine, and food and rhythm are main aspects of life—we can adjust Carrie's food and schedule to address her concerns. Nourishing her hair with herbal oils or simply avocado oil, while adding more good fats like avocado, salmon, and macadamia nuts to her diet will help correct her thinning hair. Crafting a more stable, and slower paced schedule will give her mind time to rest. And a sturdy routine will allow her mind to more organized and less forgetful. Additionally, Carrie can eat more warm and grounding foods for dinner, such as spaghetti squash and stew, for example, to ground her Vata and help help her get a complete nights sleep. The ability to identify and adjust qualities is a principle player in keeping the Doshas in a harmonious state.

Discover your Dosha and state of health via your tongue... "Open your mouth and say ahhhh". We've all had a doctor request to see our tongues. The tongue serves as an important diagnostic tool throughout many schools of medicine. Ayurveda Practitioners can get a pretty good idea of a persons constitution and health just by seeing their tongue. The shape of ones tongue helps to reveal ones constitution. Vata tongues tend to be narrow. Pitta tongues tend to be medium width and pointy, and Kapha tongues are wide and thick. The color of a persons tongue gives us information as well. When a tongue is purple, that indicates a Vata imbalance. A rich red color is indicative of heat or a Pitta imbalance, and a very pale tongue is indicative of a dim fire which lends itself to Kapha imbalances such as weak digestion and phlegm. Consistent with most visible diagnostic traits; we understand that people are complex and no single sign is necessarily absolute. Someone could have a pale tongue and great digestion. Someone else could have a very bright red tongue and be free of Pitta imbalances such as heartburn and acidity which are commonly associated with a bright red tongue. The tongue helps to give us general clues.Details on the landscape of the tongue reveal an even better picture. Ridgy edges or teeth marks around the perimeter of the tongue are consistent with malabsorption. Someone who displays this type of tongue should remove all artificial sweeteners and chemicals from their diet. Such products compromise the intestinal wall causing malabsorption. If someone has ridgy edges that look like teeth marks they can drink an Ayurvedic tea made from equal parts ginger, fennel, cumin, and coriander. This will help repair their gut health and aid in the absorption of nutrients.

Foam on the tongue can correlate with candida. Candida, a yeast like overgrowth is caused and fed by the prevalence of too much sugar in ones diet. If someone has a foamy tongue they should avoid sugar, especially while refined sugar. The Ayurvedic herbs Brahmi and Triphala are booth helpful in taking care of yeast in the body. A puffy tongue, and/or a tongue with waves along the perimeter is consistent with stagnant lymph. Eating meals too late at night, and/or drinking wine in the evening can also create a puffy tongue. People with a puffy tongue should avoid eating and drinking alcohol after sunset. These people can also try 'dry brushing' to help move the lymph. To dry brush, purchase a luffa sponge or luffa gloves and brush upwards from the base of the limbs towards the heart once daily, before a shower.

A thick coating on the tongue indicates the presence of Ama, or toxicity in the body. The location of the coating is telling as well.

A coating in the back of the tongue, near the tonsils, indicates that the toxicity is mostly in the colon. A coating in the middle of the tongue indicates that the toxins are throughout the gastrointestinal area. If someone has a thick coating on their tongue they can use a tongue scraper. A tongue scraper helps remove the topical toxins and stimulate the digestive process to prevent the build up of new toxicity. Digestive herbs such a trikatu, ginger, and triphala are all helpful in dispelling and preventing toxicity. You are now educated on the basics of tongue diagnostics. These tools can be very helpful in gathering data and keeping a gage on our personal health on a daily basis. I look at my tongue every morning, and have a habit of checking my tongue periodically throughout the day. Surveying and understanding the tongue gives us direction as to where we might need to make adjustments in with our food and supplemental routines. For example, as a Pitta/Vata constitution in a healthy state my tongue is bright pink. If I wake up and my tongue is pale, this indicates to me that my Agni, or digestive strength is weaker than usual, so I should eat lighter than usual and perhaps sip on ginger tea that day. Ayurveda is all about self-knowledge and self-healing. Your tongue is just one more place to gain insights!

Intentional Language: It is logical to name and label things to give them distinction and classification. Words hold great power, especially in our culture. The words we repeatedly hear and speak reinforce our beliefs and behaviors. For example, a little girl who is constantly being told how smart she is will foster an identity that is linked to being intelligent. In this little girl's world, her parents and teachers constantly use phrases like, "You're brilliant. You're a star student. You're so gifted." This little girl will adopt intelligence as part of her selfhood. Her automatic response to life will come from a place of believing, "I am smart". Or for instance, let us look at a little boy who is an extraordinary athlete. He is prone to winning. His room is decorated in trophies. Phrases such as, "Never give up. Failure is not an option. Give it all you've got", are in the scripts of every practice and game. This little boy will approach life with a tailored mindset fed by the language he constantly hears, believes, and replays in his mind. The language other people place on us is influential, but the language we place on ourselves is even more impactful. Returning to our positive affirmations and deliberate, "I Am" statements will help us steer the ship of where we are going. Listen to your self-talk. Observe your internal monologues. Notice how you are phrasing your current state.

The language we use can transform our experience... as a Vata I would often say, "I feel anxious." Anxious begets anxious, so in using this phrase I continued to feel more of the same, and in increasing intensity. One day it occurred to me that maybe I wasn't anxious. Maybe I was excited. When I closed my eyes, took a few deep breaths, and let my mind wander—I landed on excitement. From that day on anytime I caught myself thinking, "I am anxious", I immediately reframed the language to, "I am feeling disorganized excitement." My next thought was how can I organize this excitement? Sometimes that meant taking a bath, going on a walk, drawing up a to-do list, starting a new project, leaving my environment, or changing the topic of discussion. I realized I was able to circumvent feeling a way I didn't want to feel simply by renaming it. The language we repeatedly identify with can become the composition of a self-fulfilling prophecy. A self-fulfilling prophecy is a statement that may be initially false, but when reinforced over a period of time, by positive feedback, belief and behavior the prophecy becomes true. Be careful and compassionate with yourself when decorating yourself with labels. The conversation in your head should promote the reality you wish to partake in. Make sure whatever label you recite, and replay is something you would be happy to see more of in your life.

PAUSE FOR AFFIRMATION

"I am willing to access my best self."

Seasons Influence the Doshas: One Dosha is not better than another. We all have all three in us, just in different amounts.The proportions of our elemental makeup makes us unique. We are like snowflakes. No two alike. Factors such as season and age play a role in the presence of each Dosha in our lives. Regardless of your mind/body make up, everyone's Vata is higher in the fall because the fall is Vata's time of year. The atmospheric conditions in the fall mirror the qualities of Vata. The air is dry and rough, so the dry and rough qualities within us amplify. Have you ever noticed how your bowels become more pellet like in the fall? This is because of the dry and rough conditions. Everyone's Pitta is elevated in the summer, because the summer is Pitta's time of year. Pitta is fire and the summer is hot and humid. In such, our internal heat and moisture become magnified. Perhaps you have experienced heat rashes or acne in Mid-July. We can thank peak Pitta season for that. Likewise, everyone's Kapha is accentuated in the spring because the air is sticky and moist. Have you noticed how your allergies flare up in the spring? That is because pollen is attracted to the sticky and moist atmosphere of your sinus cavity. As a Floridian, in Florida we have two seasons at best, hot and less hot. With that, people often ask, "Well how are the Doshas effected if we don't have seasons?" Great question! The energetics of each season are perceivable to the body even if the changes in the atmosphere are not dramatic. For example, have you ever noticed how the time period between Halloween and New Years zips by? It tends to be a frenzy whirlwind of movement, shopping, festivities, exhaustion, and joy. Typically, we talk a big sigh by mid-January and think, "Whew, what just happened?" The quickening conditions of the holiday season are amplified by the qualities of Vata. Vata is light, quick, excitable, stimulated, cold and dry, as is Fall—as is Halloween through New Years. So yes, while the seasons may not be ostensible, the effects of the seasons are still captured and animated in your constitution.

Typically, if you can feel it in the atmosphere, you can feel it in the body. Have you ever been to the desert? Do you notice how your skin gets incredibly dry? Your lips lay crack and your nose might bleed. The dry quality of the desert landscape will make its way into the landscape of your body. The seasons influence our Doshic makeup because the external atmosphere replicates itself internally. An especially high amount of any one quality left to its own devices will raise the probability for a corresponding imbalance. Fall increases Vata, Summer increases Pitta, and Spring increases Kapha.

Character Sketch—Meet Spicy Christine: Pitta is a hot Dosha because it is mostly fire. The qualities of Pitta are hot, light, oily, spreading, sharp, acidic and pungent (spicy). If Christine has a predominantly Pitta constitution, she probably loves hot weather and being out in the sun (her Pitta disposition will either be attracted to, or repulsed by more heat). She has oily skin and sometimes gets acne and rashes. When she gets a rash it spreads. She is direct with his words and speaks her mind. This is all well and good, but in the summer the atmosphere is hot and the air in humid, so these like qualities will exacerbate Christine's proclivity for heat related imbalances. She is likely to become more agitated and short tempered in the summer. There's a probability that she will experience more heat related digestive complaints such as hyperacidity and heartburn during the hotter months of the year. Her skin and eyes will feel more sensitive and so on. This is essentially because in the summer she can easily pour fuel on her fire if she is not mindful.

To achieve balance: It would be advisable for Christine to stay out of the heat, and avoid spicy and acidic foods—especially in the summer. Christine would do well with shade and more cooling foods like cumber, coconut and watermelon. As a Yogi, Christine may want to reduce hot and power classes in favor of air-conditioned flow classes and yin yoga, specifically during the hotter months of the year. Christine would even enjoy a little sandalwood or lemongrass essential oil in a diffusor at the office or in her bedroom, and spritzed on her yoga mat.

> *"Man is a microcosm of the macrocosm; the God on earth is built on the pattern of God in nature."*
>
> **—Carl Jung**

Microcosm and Macrocosm: We are a microcosm of the macrocosm. We are made of the same elements as everything in the universe. From the pages of this book, to the hairs on your head, everything in the universe is constructed by shared core elements (space, air, fire, water and earth). Our patterns mimic the patterns of nature. Our digestive strength mimics the strength of the sun. Our digestion is strongest mid-day, as is the sun. Our mechanisms to restore, rest and repair mimic the cycle of the moon. Most creatures rest under the luminous lunar hours, as do we. Even our menstrual cycle mimics the cycles of the tides and moon. The ride flows in and the tide flows out.

In many ways I look at Ayurveda like a meteorologist looks at weather patterns. In reference to weather, we are familiar with terms such as moisture, dryness, wind, heat, cold, light and so on. We realize that the weather oscillates due to location, the time of day and the season. Based on science and observation we can make predictions and prepare accordingly. The mind-body system of medicine works in a similar way. We learn the qualities. We apply the science. We observe, and we formulate internal forecasts. As we learn how the season influence the Doshas, keep in mind that when it comes to qualities. The conditions of the inner world reflect the conditions of the outer world, and opposites create balance.

In the fall, the weather is cold and dry. Vata (space and air elements) will be disturbed. This will accentuate the prevalence of joints crackly, a dehydrated colon, and restless mind. We should balance these spacey and airy qualities with earth and water qualities. In the fall, we need additional warmth and oil. Eat warming foods like soups, stews, hot cereals, roasted root vegetables, and stir-fries. Use more ghee, grape seed and coconut oil when cooking. Drizzle meals with olive oil (olive oil should not get too hot because it turns rancid in extreme heat). Use oil on the body. Give yourself a loving massage with sesame oil. We use sesame oil in the fall because sesame oil has heating properties that help to keep the body warm and moisturized.

In the summer, the atmosphere is hot and damp. Pitta (fire) is provoked. This can express itself as irritation, skin inflammation and gnawing hunger. We should balance out the spicy/fire qualities with cooling summer fruits like watermelon, cantaloup and coconut. We should incorporate more water into our lives during the summer. Drink more room temperature water to rehydrate after sweating. Notice I said room temperature. Avoid the temptation to drink ice water. The freezing cold fluid shocks the body. The body doesn't thrive off extremes, so it will kick on an extra burner (aka, create extra heat) to neutralize the extreme cold you just doused it with. Avoid cold water. Even when you're hot. Play in the water. Swim, enjoy the lake and beach (wear sunscreen), bring an umbrella or scout out shade. Direct sun irritates the heck out of Pitta in the summer.

In the spring, the climate is moist and cool. Kapha (earth and water elements) will be higher than usual. This can lead to allergies, lethargy and water retention. To stay balanced in the spring, avoid mucus forming foods like dairy, sugar and wheat. Dodging dairy in the spring (or year round for that matter) will help clear your sinuses, and keep allergies at bay. Introduce local honey into your diet. Honey is a natural heating and drying agent, so it helps clear sinus congestion. Use plenty of warming spices like ginger, cayenne and black pepper to burn away congestion. Try ginger tea with a pinch of black pepper and a dash of cayenne. Bye bye congestion. Move, move, move. In spring the flowers are blossoming, animals are mating, the winter is over, and the birds are chirping. Get out and play. Be active. Activity stirs up the stagnant energy that compounds through the winter months. Move to break up stagnation, so it won't have a chance to morph into lethargy. Just as you adjust your wardrobe to accommodate for shifts in the seasons, you should also adjust your food and lifestyle to accommodate for seasonal shifts.

As a yogi, you probably have a preference for what style of yoga you tend to gravitate towards. As an Ayurvedic-Yogi you may start to adjust your practice to compliment your Doshas during seasonal transitions. During the fall and early winter, you can choose to ground your heightened Vata with warming and grounding classes such as, warm Hatha or Yin. During the Spring, you may adjust your practice to keep your Kapha harmonized by taking more invigorating classes, like Bikram, Asthanga and Heated Flow classes. These style will help break up and burn away cool mucus conditions. During the Summer months, you can quell Pitta by avoiding so many hot classes. Opt for air conditioned Flows and cooling Yin classes instead.

Age Affects the Doshas: Each Doshas rules a particular stage in our lives. Regardless of your mind-body make up, everyone's Kapha is more prevalent ages 0-20, because this is your building stage of life. Think of babies, cute little butter balls, always smiley with runny noses. Babies are more prone towards Kapha issues like colds and mucus build up. Everyone's Pitta is up between the ages of 21-50, because this is our time of ambition and acquisition. That fire drives us to achieve our goals, get our degree, house, job, spouse and so on. Everyone is more prone towards Pitta imbalances like acne and irritation during the Pitta stage of life. Then around age 51, we reach a new stage of life, ”The Wisdom Years”. In this stage of life our Vata is higher, because not working so much allows our schedules to be more flexible, our sleep and digestion lighten up, and we feel called to tap into our intuition and insight to discover deeper meaning, and the purpose for our lives. Everyone is more prone toward Vata imbalances like forgetfulness and insomnia during the Vata stage of life. To become aware of the probability for specific imbalances in a specific stages of life is not to alarm us, but to prepare us. We can sidestep imbalances by fostering our awareness, attitudes and actions to compensate for the organic junctures of life. And should we encounter an imbalance, we can treat the imbalance as an opportunity to learn and grow.

> *"When you don't come across any problems, you can be sure that you are traveling the wrong path."*
>
> **—Swami Vivekananda**

An imbalance is not a flaw or curse. Imbalances are signs of life. I love Tony Robbins who says, "Problems are signs of life." Life would be boring if everything was always the same. We require a certain sense of certainty (for example, the sun will come up tomorrow), however we also require a healthy sense of variety. It is in our design to be in a state of fluctuation. Fluctuation provides variety, and variety is the gestation area for growth. The body is very smart. We are programed for vacillations of imbalance and balance. The concern occurs only when we have missed a volume of glaring signs and signals that we have abandoned our True Nature. (Remember, we want to hear the whisper so we don't have to deal with the scream). Pay attention to qualities; qualities function as signals. Balance qualities by introducing the opposite. Too much heat? Add cooling items. It's quite simple.

> *"Practice and all is coming."*
>
> **—Sri K. Pattabhi Jois**

Just Like Yoga, Ayurveda is a Daily Practice... Your yoga tool box may include a mat, blocks, a strap, a studio you call home, a breathing and or meditation practice, a tribe of fellow yogis, a video, a set of intentions, an inspiring teacher,and a series of invigorating and relaxing postures. You count on these tools. You may not use them everyday or all at once, but you have them. You know they're loyal, accessible and effective. Ayurveda comes with tools too, in fact yoga is one of the tools. We call it "Yoga Chakitsa", or yoga therapy. In your toolbox you will also find healthful food, balanced daily rhythms, movement in nature, meditation, breathing practices, spices, herbs, essential oils, and self-care routines.

Sturdy schedules and grounding routines provide remarkable benefits for Vata types. Due to my constitution and lifestyle, I have a tendency to become Vata imbalanced. Not long ago, I was in the midst of moving offices, as well as simultaneously moving into a new home. My days were bursting at the seams with teaching, seeing clients, packing, and trying to juggle social engagements, all while trying to complete this book. Half of my belongings were in storage, my old apartment was entirely packed up, and I was living out of a suitcase. In efforts to keep the kitchen clean I was eating mostly quick and convenient raw food off paper plates. Untethered variables and mobs of moving parts had officially taken over. This created my most severe Vata imbalance I'd ever consciously experienced. My Vata was blowing with vengeance. I was anxious, exhausted, forgetful, constipated, and suffering from intense gas and stomach pains. I have a high pain threshold, but one day the pain was agonizing enough to call a friend who is a nurse practitioner to rule out appendicitis. I remember the distinct moment appendicitis was ruled out and my lightbulb turned on and said, "Kristen, your Vata is out of control. Sit down. Slow down. Relax." I then took a deep breath. I lied on the bed and did, "wind relieving pose," this is where you pull your knee into your chest and breathe (in case you are wondering, it works). I relieved some wind, which is excess Vata. I made a commitment to hit pause on my chaotic agenda, and return to everything I know to be true and helpful. Using the tools I am sharing with you in this book, I successfully restored my sanity and wellbeing over the course of the following weeks. I share this with you because just because we know something, does not mean we always practice it. Life happens. I certainly did not become infatuated with Ayurveda because I was already balanced and perfectly healthy. My fondness for Ayurveda grew because I needed it. I needed tools to help me find balance, and feel comfortable in my body. Ayurveda taught me to help myself, which I knew to be necessary if I wanted to help anyone else. Irrespective of your Dosha, take care to ground your Vata because in today's quick moving world it can become elevated in assiduous ways. When you're feeling, "off", but you have a lot to take care of—dial back to these simple tools, and take care of yourself first.

"Simplicity is the ultimate sophistication."

—Leonardo da Vinci

A big portion of becoming healthier has less to do with what you add in and more to do with what you subtract. This may include unnecessary stressors like unhealthy relationships, disheartened pursuits, and erratic schedules, as well as unhealthy food, chemicals, and stimulants. The idea of less is more reminds me of a this little story; A young boy watched an artist sketch a picture of a horse. The horse looked to flawless, realistic and breathtaking. Every contour and detail, down to the hairs on the mane and lashes around the eyes were absolute perfection. The little boys asked the artist, "How are you able to draw such a outstanding horse?" The artist replied, "Simple, I erase everything that's not horse." To begin, scan your life, see if there are variables that are doing more harm than good. The first step is recognizing what variables are enhancing your health and happiness, and by contrast—which ones may be detracting from health and happiness? Can you take the initial steps to reduce or remove variables that are not "horse"? Removing what we don't need creates more space for the aspects we do need to thrive. Celebrate what is adding value, but do not condemn yourself for the things that need improvement. All shifts start with understanding. You are collecting information and fortifying your sense of understanding. You do not need to "do" anything yet. The awareness is enough. Ask yourself this question: What in my life right now is adding value, and what in my life right now is not?

PAUSE FOR AFFIRMATION

"I am attracting into my life people who align with the highest ideals of myself."

Homeostasis is balance. The body is brilliant and has every capacity to auto correct, realign and heal. I love this quote by Deepak Chopra, who is one of the world's leaders in the field of mind-body medicine. He says, "The body will heal, we just need not interfere." Homeostasis is the body's tendency towards a relative and stable equilibrium between elements. Homeostasis is balance. Our body wants to be in homeostasis. Like Deepak says, "We need not interfere." How often are we tired, but rather than sleeping like the body would suggest, we interfere by gulping a coffee to force ourselves to get more done before we allow ourselves to rest? I know I've done it. Plenty. What about when we're hungry, and the body requests nourishment, but we interfere with that signal because we're too busy or we've decided to be restrictive that day? These are very basic examples on how we interfere. We live in an incredible era of instant. Instant communication, instant gratification, instant food even instant sharing through immediate Facebook updates and Instagram. Instant isn't always better. Like the old saying,"Rome wasn't built in a day," great things take time. Healing can happen spontaneously, other times healing requires patience. It is in our design to be in balance. The course in miracles says, "Patience comes naturally to those who trust." Trust yourself. Trust your capacity to be in balance. Trust the flow of life as it guides you. If you have strayed from homeostasis, be patient—you will wander back.

> *"Happiness is not a matter of intensity, but of balance, order, rhythm and harmony."*
>
> **—Thomas Merton**

Giving ourselves the time and space to organically return to our True Nature requires patience. Patience is fruitful virtue. As you embark on your journey be kind, and consistent with yourself. As an Ayurvedic wellness counselor, I interchangeable call my clients friends because to me, that is what they are. We are all navigating through this human experience, and the more good people you can have on your team, the better. Recently, I had a friend sitting across from me at the consultation table, she relayed her tale of how she does very well following all the suggestions, gets into a groove and feels better. But after a short time, she falls off the wagon, slips back into her old ways, and feels like she's slid backwards and backed into 'zero' again (a Vata tendency.) My friend's definition of zero was not flattering. I sat there looking at a woman who I knew to be strong, motivated and astute. I empathized with her tendency to create expectations for herself, and feel frustrated when the followthrough doesn't progress as planned. I expressed to her that every time she goes back to zero, as she calls it, she is going back with a new awareness. She revisits a new starting point each time with a deeper sense of self-knowledge, therefore her zero never remains zero. Zero keeps bumping up to one, two, three and so on. Over time, she continues to meet her fresh starting points with a broader perspective, as the result of her experiences and growth. This realization made her smile. I believe this to be true for all of us. Our setbacks don't set us back. They create new platforms to help us move forward.

> *"Our greatest glory is not in never failing, but in rising every time we fall."*
>
> **—Confucius**

> **Practice:** *Make a list of aspects of your life that are strengthening your wellbeing. Perhaps yoga, good friends, journaling, a project you enjoy ect. In contrast, make a list of aspects of your life that may be weakening your wellbeing. Perhaps, saying yes to engagements you'd rather not attend, not preparing meals at home, maybe an over indulgence of wine or coffee, or skipping meditation because you're in a hurry.*

How the Doshas Influence Our Relationships... Whether you love them, avoid them, or cherish them, we all have them. We have relationships with our food, ourselves, our jobs, kids, environments, and partners to name a few. Every interaction and encounter is by some definition a relationship. Who of us has not glanced through articles, magazines, blogs, and books with a hungry curiosity for ways to strengthen, distance, protect, or correct our ties and bonds? Ayurveda offers us intriguing and telling secrets into the dynamic workings of our relationships. According to Ayurveda there are three pillars of health: food, sex, and sleep. The three greatest categories of wellbeing engulf our lives through the qualities of nutrition we consume, the lifestyle we chose, and the relationships we entertain. While attending Ayurveda school I was decorated with a piece of advice that has not left my side, "for good health, eat good food, and keep good company." Simple and profound. Of the multitude of things we expose ourselves to, are forced to digest, assimilate, and eliminate, relationships have arguably the greatest impact on our wellbeing. As we brushed upon, the three mind-body constitutions sum up three distinctive, but not limiting categories of personalities. Vata types, composed of mostly the air element are creative, active, intuitive, spontaneous, expressive and adaptable. Pitta personalities, composed of plenty of fire element are ambitious, goal oriented, charismatic, competitive, sharp, leader types. And Kaphas, who are mostly earth element tend to be grounded, go with the flow, mellow, loyal, sweet, reliable and nurturing. The processes and progression of civilization rely heavily upon on a diverse and colorful playground. As a kid my dad always said, "It takes all kinds to make the world go round." While existence on a day to day basis functions thanks to a wide range of similarities and dichotomies in personality types, you probably prefer to spend more time with people you are intrinsically compatible with. There is an advantage to knowing your nature and tendencies, as well as gathering a basic understanding of the nature and tendencies of the person or people you are closest to. In relationships, If you are a Vata type, or find yourself doughy eyed and smitten for one, perhaps you should be aware of the instinctual patterns known to Vatas. Vatas tend to get anxious, worried, insecure, forgetful, whimsical, a bit scattered, or unfocused in times of stress and instability. Treat Vatas like a butterfly. These people are delicate (This is different from fragile. They are not easily broken, but like the wings of a butterfly. They are sensitive to their surroundings). Vatas need a dose of reassuring, predictability, and structure in relationships. These quick moving little beings respond well to someone who gives a firm touch, makes decisions, but provides space for their wings to spread as needed. Do not cage a Vata in with overly strict schedules and tight agendas. Within a sensible structure, they need freedom for spontaneity and creative whims. Vata types will get anxious, fleet or retract if you are forceful and pushy, or conversely, distant and unreliable. Vatas are balanced by more even tempered mannerisms and actions. Likewise, if you are in a relationship with a Vata, do not to be wishy-washy. Vata types appreciate a stable loyal place to land each day. Vatas do well with someone who can help ground them. To win the heart of a Vata surprise them with a creative and spontaneous date. Then give them a relaxing foot massage. The creativity contrasts with the grounding massage to create a perfectly balanced day.Pittas. Fiery friends and lovers of fiery friends—caution. You are playing with fire. Pittas are all things passionate and charming. Pittas need to be with someone they respect. Treat a Pitta like a partner, a comrade, and a teammate. Pittas do well with intellectual stimulation, direct/sensual touch, and collaborative journeys towards a shared goal. Pittas might get irritated by flighty/unfocused behaviors, as well as lazy/complacent behaviors. This is because they are remarkably driven. Pittas typically want to excel in whatever they do, and relationships are not excluded. In relationships, Pittas should be mindful not to compete with their partners. Co-creating would be a better option. Pittas are soothed by water activities and sweet flowers. So, if you love a Pitta invite flowers and cool blue colors into your romantic and living spaces. Provide serene atmospheres that welcome time to unwind and refresh together. Kaphas tend to be like teddy bears. These snuggle types love romance with an affinity towards all things sweet and nurturing. If you are dating a Kapha, expect to be taken care of with delicious meals, or provided for with financial cushioning. Kaphas are providers and caretakers at heart. They gravitate towards relaxed dates like movies, long dinners, and nights curled up by the fireplace. Kaphas can benefit from the sprightly nature if a Vata or heated motivation of a Pitta to get them moving. To win the heart if a Kapha, play on the sentimental acts of affection. Make them a scrapbook, give them sweet kisses, a home made desert, or hand written card (the will keep it forever.) There is no one said correct combination. We can do not neatly fit into perfect little boxes marked, Vata, Pitta, and Kapha. Relationships are not calculated algorithms. Relationships are built on the basis of love, experience, and willingness to grow. Together. As the adage goes, "Where there is love, there is a way". I believe people are placed in our lives for a reason. If we have a chemistry or connection with someone, an opportunity to learn and develop is certainly in the design. But by peeking at yourself and your partner through this perspective you will find yourself more accepting, appreciative, and even savvy in the ways you navigate this messy, complicated, exhilarated, rewarding, and necessary arena of life. Keep in mind Vatas tend to be sporadic. Regarding relationships Vatas can confuse an unknowing heart because they can be very excited one minute then withdrawn the next. Because of their adaptable nature, Vatas are resilient to quick and fleeting relationships. But do not be fooled these little bodies hold big hearts, and when the time comes they too can settle down. (Just take them on vacation so they do not get antsy.) Pittas tend to pour a lot of fuel onto the fire of their hearts.

Do not be intimidated by the intensity of a Pitta suitor. Pittas are analytical, and will likely weigh the pros and cons, potentials, and red flags early on. A Pitta will not waste their time nor yours. When a Pitta finds his/her match, bring your hose and get ready for an adventure. Kaphas are the most loyal of the three. With an aversion to change these snuggly creatures are slow to fall in love, but once they do it will last. If you are craving the sweetness of a Kapha be patient, they will come around.

> *"Your task is not to seek for love, but merely to seek and find all the barriers within yourself you have build against it."*
>
> **—Course in Miracles**

An Outlined Reference for Identifying the Doshas and Achieving Balance

Balanced Vata

PHYSICAL CHARACTERISTICS	EMOTIONAL CHARACTERISTICS
thin, light frame	loves excitement and new experiences
irregular appetite and digestion	quick to anger and quick to forgive
dry skin	energetic
cold hands and feet	creative
loves movement	adaptable

Imbalanced Vata

PHYSICAL IMBALANCES	EMOTIONAL IMBALANCES
weight loss	prone to worry
constipation	anxiety
gas and bloating	insomnia
hypertension	forgetfulness
arthritis	overwhelmed
weakness	stressed

The ABCs of Balancing Vata

Slow down
Create a stable routine
Don't skip meals
Remove excess stimulus (too much screen time: TV, computer, gadgets ect.)
Drink ginger tea to support digestion (Detox & Replenish Tea by Wellblends)
Take special care in the Fall
Avoid excess cold and raw foods
Use lavender, chamomile, ylang ylang and sweet orange organic essential oils to ground and relax

Balanced Pitta

PHYSICAL CHARACTERISTICS	EMOTIONAL CHARACTERISTICS
medium size and weight	powerful intellect
bright red hair, fine hair, or grey or balding hair	good concentration
excellent digestion, strong appetite	good decision makers
warm body temperature	good leaders, teachers and speakers
lustrous complexion	driven
abundant energy	witty

Imbalanced Pitta

PHYSICAL IMBALANCES	EMOTIONAL IMBALANCES
skin rashes, acne, blemishes	aggressive/overly competitive
burning sensations	judgmental
excessive body heat	short-tempered
indigestion, heart burn	argumenative
peptic ulcers	arrogant

The ABCs of Balancing Pitta

Do not over work. Do—schedule down time
Do not skip meals
Spend time in nature
Drink cooling tea like fennel, cumin and coriander
Favor cooling colors like blue and green
Take special care in the summer
Avoid spicy and acidic foods
Use lemon, peppermint, sandalwood, rose and fennel organic essential oils to refresh.

Balanced Kapha

PHYSICAL CHARACTERISTICS	EMOTIONAL CHARACTERISTICS
strong build	calm
excellent stamina	thoughtful
large eyes	loyal
soft and smooth skin	patient
thick and voluminous hair	steady, supportive
sound sleep	committed
slower digestion	nurturing

Imbalanced Kapha

PHYSICAL IMBALANCES	EMOTIONAL IMBALANCES
weight gain	lethargic
fluid retention	depressed
allergies	greedy
excessive sleep	jealous
asthma	resistant to change
diabetes	stubborness

The ABCs of Balancing Kapha

Seek stimulation—new sights, activities and experiences
Wake up early and avoid naps
Drink heating teas to stimulate digestion, like ginger, clove and cinnamon
Make exercise a priority
Take special care in the spring
Avoid heavy and mucus forming foods like sugar, wheat and dairy
Use eucalyptus, basil, camphor, clove, and lemon organic essential oils to rejuvenate.

CHAPTER THREE

Explore Health

"Samadosha, samagnischa, samadhatumala, kriyaha prasanna atmenindriya manaha swasthya itybhidheeyate."

—Sushruta

"Health is a state where the three Doshas, digestive fire, all the bodily tissues and components, and all the physiological processes are in perfect unison. Health is when the soul, sense organs, and mind are all in a state of total satisfaction and contentment."

OUR CURRENT HEALTH care model subscribes to the idea that if we are not sick, we must be healthy. Health is more than being free from disease. Health is the harmonious state where the body, mind and soul function in trinity with one another. Health is not something we fight to achieve. Disease is not something we attack. Health is found in the presence of peace. As we actively engage self-confidence, and employ intuitive strategies to keep our day to day wellbeing in our own hands, we forge a path for redefining health, as not the absence of disease, but the complete presence of life.

> *"The state of health is a moment to moment happening. Healing is moment to moment balance, brining awareness to our thoughts, feelings and emotions and how we respond."*
>
> **—Vasant Lad**

Disease quite literally means the disconnect from ease. The word Disease and the combination of two words Dis, as in disconnect and Ease, as in harmony. The call to heal is not a call to attack. Fighting creates the atmosphere of conflict. Conflict is the opposite of ease. To heal we need to bridge the gap. We need to counterbalance a disease by inviting in more ease. All Disease is the bodies request to dismiss the agents of harm, and invite in the agents of peace. I know this may sound funny, but this is how we end war on a very personal level. I don't know if you have ever fought yourself, but I spent years being at war with myself. I wanted my body to be something different from what it was. I pushed it, starved it, ignored it, disliked it, the list goes on. These actions made me sprint further away from my True Nature. Fast. In such, I didn't feel excellent. It wasn't until I started to first acknowledge my body, begin to accept it, listen to it, love it and finally treat it like I loved it, that I began to truly feel embody ease. Interestingly enough, once I felt at ease with my body, the absence of disease became conventional. I rarely get sick, and when I do I appreciate the sickness as my bodies way of encouraging me to slow down, pay attention and take care. Wayne

Dyer says, "What you resist persists." If we are always thinking about what we don't want (to be sick, fat, tired, lonely, broke, you name it), we will continue to see the presence of the very thing we resist endure in our lives. For instance, if you've ever been on a diet, you're familiar with the torturous experience of thinking about food all day long. Food is the one thing you're supposed to be limiting, and consuming less of, yet the restriction actually has you daydreaming of everything you "can't" have, and salivating more so than if you were not on the diet. What we resists persists.

Healing requests that we focus on, and bring forth more of what we want in our lives, and for our health. Peace cannot come from war. If we are in a state of disease, concentrating our attention on the disease by means of attack will not make us feel better. A person near and dear to my heart recently passed as the ultimate result of cancer. She was a magnificent woman, with more creativity, kindness and generosity in her five-foot frame than anyone I had ever met. During the final years of her life the word cancer had become the most dominant word in her vocabulary and one of the most readily spoken upon topics in her day to day conversations with loved ones, care takers and new friends. Health care professionals often refer to the process of overcoming cancer as, "The war on cancer." Her life became consumed by chemotherapy, doctors appointments and explicit schedules of when to take pills and drink specific fluids. Throughout the course of, "Fighting cancer," she was an embodiment of strength and courage. In the end, cancer overcame her physical body. I will always admire her, for her grace and perseverance were robust. We cannot ignore that which inundates our lives, especially when the visceral pain inhibits or ability to do ordinary things like comfortably eat, go for walks or even take a shower. Each of us must chart our own path. We are entitled to our own curiosities, explorations, and beliefs. How we choose to approach anything in our lives is like everything in our lives—deeply personal. I just can't help but wonder what I would do in that scenario. Would choosing to surround myself with health, by bringing flowers into my room, only consuming organic fruits and vegetables, forbidding any talk of sickness, plastering my walls with photographs and images that sparked happiness, becoming absorbed in inspiring books and podcasts, surrounding myself with loved ones, and meditating on healing be enough to change the course of such a trajectory? I do not have these answers. At this point, I only have these questions. Perhaps there are certain trajectories that are laid in place by a grander dream maker, where the invisible echo of purpose, reason and time are imperceptible by these particular human eyes on this particular mortal plane. Perhaps, some things are not meant to be dismantled or re-written. But, for as long as we get to author our own scripts to whatever degree—I think we owe it to ourselves to honor our beliefs, whatever they may be with grace and dignity. What I do know is, for the final weeks of her life, all my wonderful loved one wanted to do was be in the comfort of her own home. Home is where health begins, and sometimes it may come full circle to where it ends. Wherever we are in sickness or health, may we always be surrounded by love. Irrespective of beliefs, I do not know a single person who cannot benefit from love. In many ways, love is highly medicinal.

"Embrace uncertainty. Some of the most beautiful chapters in our lives won't have titles until much later."

—Bob Goff

Disease is the absence of ease. I understand that some of you are reading this now thinking, "Look Honey, I have a catalog of blood work, lab reports, mammograms, pap smears and cat scans, and the like that indicate I'm in some serious trouble. I don't know if a little more ease is going to get me out of this mess." I understand. There are cases where the condition is too pressing for Ayurvedic principles and self-care techniques to be your stand alone form of medicine. In this case it will benefit you to allow the system of Ayurveda to cushion and support you while you continue other forms of treatment. No matter what the condition, it seems irrefutable to me that awareness, balance, self-care, and nourishment will at the very least illicit the mechanisms for self-healing.

> *"Whenever you take an adversarial attitude toward something, you give it power."*
>
> **—Christine Northcrup**

The Application. Use Opposites to Create Balance. We live in a universe of dualities. Angels and demons, day and night, male and female, happy and sad, yin and yang. Go on, compile a list of opposites. It's entertaining. At first glance it might seem like a clashing pile of juxtapositions, but within the disorder, there is always order. The law of opposites states that when you approach an imbalance, you should spot the quality of provocation and apply the opposite to create balance. It's as simple as when you walk into a dark room, it will remain dark. Now walk into a dark room while carrying a flash light and the room has light. This is balance. For example, if someone is suffering from hypothermia—the person is extremely cold. If you apply heat, you create balance.

If someone is burning up with a fever, and apply cold socks to their feet, and a cold compress to their forehead, you create balance. If someone's skin is hot, flaky and itchy—you can apply cool, moisturizing, and soothing coconut oil to create balance. If someone has acid reflux, you give them an acid neutralizer like fenugreek capsules or water with baking soda. It is simple, relatively intuitive, and effective.

> *"Darkness can not drive out darkness, only light can do that. Hate can not drive out hate, only love can do that."*
>
> **—Martin Luther King**

Surround a disease with health. This applies to many facets of life. Surround suffering with compassion, surround despair with hope, surround hostility with peace, and surround fear with trust. The principal tool in Ayurveda is that, "Like creates more like" and, "Opposites create balance". If you are sick, do not focus on sick; focus on health. Focus on solutions. If you are sad, don't let sad consume you; see where you can entertain joy. In you are in an adverse state, give yourself permission to allow the opposite experience to present itself. If you are so stuck on the current experience, you create a barrier between you and a new experience. Surrounding adversity with positivity is a craft. There is an art to balance.

Taking a nuanced look at the qualities, and applying opposites to shift the Doshas back into balance… Similar to the example with my friend Carrie, if someone has a Vata imbalance that means there are too many light, dry, rough, quick and cold qualities governing. So we will add in heavy, moist, slow, warm and oily through foods and lifestyle. In the case of a Pitta imbalance, there are too many hot, sharp, oily, light and spreading qualities. We'll apply cool, dry, heavy and stable qualities. For a Kapha imbalance, there are too many heavy, cool, dull, slow, sticky, stable and slimy qualities; we'll apply light, sharp, quick, dry and rough qualities.

> *"Anyone who believes that anything can be suited to everyone is a great fool, because medicine is practiced not on mankind in general, but on every individual in particular."*
>
> **—Henri de Mondeville**

Character Sketch: Meet Emily: Emily is thin. Her hair and skin are dry and rough. Emily loves running. She currently in college, on the track team, and works part time at a pizza place. Her schedule is busy and demanding. Emily typically just eats quick snack bars and smoothies because she doesn't have time to cook. Emily hates the fall because she feels so cold and her joints hurt when she runs. The same dry qualities that appear in her skin and hair are also present in her joints, digestive tract, and elimination channels. The dryness in her joints cause popping and cracking. The dryness and roughness in her digestive tract and elimination channels cause gas, bloating, constipation and dry-pellet like stools. Emily has a Vata imbalance.

Shifting Emily into Balance: We bring Emily balance by introducing opposites. The opposite of light is heavy and the opposite of cold is hot. So we will encourage Emily to swap out those cold and light foods, (like snack bars and smoothies) for warmer and heavier foods. She can easily make soups in a crock pot or grab a bowl of chili or stew from a cafe. Rather than eating cold packaged snack bars, she can eat hot oatmeal with dates and cinnamon. That will help, but let's look at a few more of Emily's dominate qualities. The opposite of quick is slow, and the opposite of dry is oily or moist. Emily loves to run and she rushes from one activity to the next. It may be advisable for Emily to reduce her number of days at the pizza joint. She may be able to work fewer days, but more hours when she's there. This will save her from crowding everyday with the extra clutter of getting ready for work, driving to work, walking around for a few hours at work and driving home. That is a lot of unnecessary movement. If it is impossible for Emily to change her work schedule, we can have her counterbalance some of that movement with stillness. When she arrives to work she can pause and ground with a few deep breaths in her car before rushing in. When she gets home she can ground with a stable nightly routine like a few restorative yoga postures and a quieting meditation. Stillness is the opposite of movement, and will inherently incite balance in the life of a busy Vata. Emily loves running, so I wouldn't nudge her to necessarily stop something she loves, but she could balance out the quickness of running by following it up with something very slow such as a hot bath, or a few restorative yoga poses. It would be life changing for Emily to wake up 10 minutes earlier everyday to meditate. During that 10 minutes she could sit up, take a few deep breaths, watch her breaths, and listen to soothing music before getting ready. Meditation is calming. It promotes an inner tranquility that will serve as a buffer for her quick movements later in the day. Emily tends to be dry. As mentioned, the opposite of dry is moist or oily. Emily can add more moisture into her body by drinking more warm water (it is more hydrating that cold water). She can eat more moist foods like soups, root vegetables (like sweet potatoes and yams), and enjoy dates as a snack. Nothing counter balances dryness quite like oil. I would suggest that Emily use coconut oil and ghee when cooking. I would advise Emily to rub oil on her body every night, especially in the fall (Vata season). Oil is smooth and hydrating. Oil is far more effective than lotion in counter balancing dry and rough qualities because it soothes beyond the skin. It saturates deeply and calms the nervous system. These qualities of sesame oil would be the best oil for Emily because sesame oil is heavy and warming. By applying these measures, Emily will notice that her joints feel better, her skin and hair feel healthier, and her bowels are more regular. The cherry on top is that she will be universally, more calm. You can see here, that this treatment plan does not require any pill bottles.The treatment plans Ayurveda offers us are not extreme or invasive; they adhere to an individuals already established life in a way that reduces chaos and brings harmony for the mind-body.

Pittas easily become too hot, oily, sharp, and light, so we remedy with cool, dry, and a more even tempered food and lifestyle to achieve balance.

Character Sketch: Meet Alex: Alex is an attorney. Her days are long and demanding. Alex has always been a competitive athlete, so even though she doesn't compete anymore, exercise is very important to her. She wakes up at 7am to drink coffee, then run on the treadmill. She takes a hot shower, swings through Starbucks for another dose of caffeine, and blazes into the office for days jam packed with meetings and paperwork. Alex usually doesn't have much time for lunch, so she orders in Chinese or Thai food. She loves food with a kick. She often attends cocktail parties and after dinner meetings with clients and associates. It is not out of character for Alex to let her hair down with several clicks of a martini glass.

To bring Alex balance we need to introduce opposites. The most prevailing qualities in Alex are hot, light, sharp, pungent (spicy) and oily. The opposite of hot is cold. I would suggest that Alex make a few adjustments in her daily routine. Alex could easily swap her early morning coffee for warm water with lemon. Coffee is very heating and acidic, and because of Alex's strong Pitta disposition, she is already hot and acidic. Warm water with lemon is far less heating than coffee, and will help alkalize her body and restore her micro-biome (gut health). Being alkaline means the body is PH balanced, this is exactly what we need to contrast acidity. By becoming alkaline, possible acidity issues like inflammation, heartburn and acid reflux will subside. After Alex runs, she may prefer a warm shower verses burning hot shower. I would suggest she put a dash of cardamom in her coffee when she swings through Starbucks. Cardamom is a spice that helps reduce acidity and helps us metabolize caffeine. Once Alex is at work, I would strongly encourage her to pause—step away from her work, and take a few deep breaths periodically. She would benefit from sipping room temperature water throughout the day. This will soften her tendency to bulldoze through her days. I would advise her to order her food that is less spicy, and snack on sweet fruits, like fresh melon, and coconut shavings. Sweetness counterbalances spicy because the opposite of spicy is sweet. Adding sweet foods such as apples, berries, figs, carrots, and watermelon slices will help compliment Alex's personality and behaviors. She will notice that she's less impatient, and her tendency to become irritable will drastically reduce if she assuages her hot tendencies. Because Alex has an inclination to function from the territories of hot and sharp, I would encourage Alex to close out her days with coolness and sweetness. She should rub a thin layer of coconut oil over her skin, because coconut oil is cool and sweet. She could take extra care to really knead and massage into the soles of her feet to relieve tension. Alex could then lie in bed and sip sweet rose, or chamomile tea to totally unwind. These minor adjustments would make a world of difference in the way Alex thinks and feels. Her body would be very grateful too. Pittas may be hesitant to become calmer and cooler in fear that they may become less efficient and productive. This is not so. Becoming balanced will reduce the likelihood of burning out. Balance promotes and prolongs efficiency and productivity.

"A person can achieve everything by being simple and humble."

—Rig Veda

Little changes have the capacity to create dramatic shifts. I realize these suggestions seem simple, we must not trivialize the value of simplicity. I am sharing these principles from a shared human experience that encapsulates a broad spectrum of limitations, possibilities, highs and lows. We all go through waves. Time and time again, I find that these principles help modulate the extremes of life.

Now let's look at Kapha: People with a strong Kapha constitution or imbalance have too many cold, damp, slow, heavy, sticky qualities, so integrating warmer, dryer and quicker/lighter foods and activities will help create balance.

Character Sketch: Meet Sarah: Sarah is nurse practitioner and mother of three. She's always caring for someone, and in turn her own self-care tends to take a back seat. She loves her patients and her family, but often feels heavy and tired throughout the day, and certainly run down by the days end. Sarah starts her day with a latte. She make the kid's lunches and grabs a bagel or muffin as she heads out. She spends all day at the doctor's office, and usually skips lunch. For dinner, time is of the essence, so it is common for Sarah to make a big vat of pasta, or macaroni and cheese for she and her family.

Now let's overlay a few modifications into Sarah's day, so that she feels better. Sarah's dominant Dosha qualities are heavy, dull, slow, sticky, thick and cold. All dairy products are heavy, dull, slow, sticky, thick and cold. Look at cheese for example, it's heavy, thick, cold and slow to digest.You can feel these qualities when you touch it or consume it. I would suggest Sarah swap her latte for a regular coffee, with a splash of almond milk. Because Sarah experiences typical Kapha imbalances like congestion and weight gain, I would recommend that Sarah add a dash of cinnamon to her coffee. Cinnamon is warming and warming spices help burn away congestion and rev-up ones metabolism. Sarah could exchange her love for coffee for a new affection for ginger tea with a pinch of clove. These heating agents will boost her metabolism. I respect how much Sarah adores her family and patients, but I would encourage her to demonstrate the same amount of care for herself too. Taking the time to eat lunch is essential. Our digestion is strongest mid-day, so Sarah would benefit from eating at lunchtime so that she doesn't overeat at night when her digestion is innately slower. Sarah could easily bring a bowl of soup or a tossed salad drizzled with a little bit of warm oil (to wilt the leafy greens) to work with her. The extra fifteen minutes it takes to mindfully eat a light and nutritious meal with be well worth her time. When Sarah returns home to her family, I would suggest that she makes a big plate of sautéed or roasted vegetables, along with her usual recipe for her kids. She should allow the vegetables to consume the majority of her plate, that way she is filling up on light foods. Light is the opposite of heavy, so that will bring Sarah into balance. Sarah has a tendency towards slowness or sluggishness, so movement is medicine for Sarah. She could do a few sun salutations after work or take a stroll after dinner. Remember one of the qualities of Kapha Dosha is slow, so a little rhythmic or rapid movement is the perfect counter balance for Sarah.

> *"The secret of change is to focus all of your energy, not on fighting the old, but building the new."*
>
> **—Socrates**

Approaching Change: Some of these changes might seem like a no-brainer, while others will require more initial thought, discipline, and effort. For best results, we want to approach balance with balance. Try not to be rigid or extreme. Follow your intuition. We do not want to completely flip our routines and habits upside down, (even if we now realize they're not serving us) because a rapid 180 like that could throw us further off kilter. Quick and drastic changes in habits do not historically last very long. Generally, slow and steady changes create lasting and sustainable patterns. Your constitution will influence how you approach change. Vata types are quick to make changes. They get very excited and do everything right away, but then they lose interest and focus. It would be wise for a Vata to slow down and integrate changes day by day. Try not to do too much all at once, this can be overwhelming for a Vata. A slow and steady approach will provide an opportunity to deeply integrate the change at the level of foundation.

> *"Everyone starts as a beginner. There is no rush. Build something that is solid instead of fast and shiny."*
>
> **—Kathryn Budig**

Pittas will decide to make changes once they've gathered all the facts. Once they make the deliberate decision, they will organize a plan and stick to it. Pittas want to be good at their new plan. It is important for Pittas to remember that their plan should also be enjoyable and have room for flexibility. Pittas should be friendly in their approach. This is not a competition, (with yourself or others). Perfection is not the goal. The aim is balance. Kapha types are the most resistant to change. Kaphas will need more consistent motivation and encouragement to get the ball rolling. Once Kaphas settle into a new healthy routine that they enjoy, they will remain loyal to it. Kapha types will benefit from building a support team to help support their path and hold them accountable. I have a client named Melissa who is Kapha. She felt a strong impulse and need to workout constantly. She expressed a concern for not having someone to keep her motivated and to hold her accountable, so I volunteered to message her every morning. I sent her silly pictures of babies doing one armed planks and Richard Simmons dancing. Daily motivation is helpful for Kaphas to keep their momentum alive.

> *"Change is hard at first, messy in the middle and gorgeous at the end."*
>
> **—Robin Sharma**

I love this phrase by Dr. Lad, who one of the most revered Ayurvedic physicians on the planet. He says, "Treat Vatas like a flower, Pittas like a peer, and Kaphas like an enemy." What he means is, Vatas are delicate and sensitive. We should be grounded and soft with Vata types. Pittas want to be in the presence of equals. Pittas will not respect you if you allow them to walk all over you, and will spite you if you are condescending towards them. Kapha types are so lovely and ooey-gooey, so we have to be a bit more direct and commanding to get their attention and motivate change. I am reminded of these character traits when i'm working with clients. I always remind my Vata friends too slow down, my Pitta friends not to take it too seriously by focusing on the details and missing the big picture, and I encourage my Kapha friends to take more initiative and be proactive. Move with gusto. Notice how you approach change, and remind yourself to incorporate the opposite of your usual tendencies to create balance. If you're doing too much, too fast—slow down and simplify. If you're competing with yourself and are steadfast on perfection—lighten up on yourself and bring in a sense of experiment and playfulness. If you're struggling to get started and feel a bit stuck—jump up and move. As Nike proudly says, "Just do it!". Your approach should be customized for you.

PAUSE FOR AFFIRMATION

"I am balanced."

"All that exists in the heavens rests in the control of Prana. As a mother of children, oh Prana, protect us, and give us splendor, and wisdom."

—Prashna Upanishad 11.13

PRANA…Increase the Good Stuff: As you may have noticed, I resonate with the idea of adding in enormous amounts of good stuff so that there simply isn't room for anything else. Scientists are doing research where they drown out destructive cells by flushing so many nutrients, antioxidants, and immune boosting agents into the body that the destructive cells cannot survive in such a thriving atmosphere. The ability to thrive is largely dependent on the presence of Prana. As a Yogi, you may be familiar with the term Prana. Prana is our life force, or chi (pronounced chee, the Chinese Medicine term for the same vital energy). It is the energy that drives life. Our breath is the ultimate source of Prana. Without breath, there is no life. Other forms of Prana can be found in nature and nutrient-rich whole foods. Ayurveda teaches us, "Follow the Prana and you will destroy the disease. Follow the disease and you will destroy the Prana." If we view disease as a call to attack, (often times with chemicals and invasive measures) we may eradicate the disease, but at the determinant of desecrating the energy that give us the power to thrive. Conversely, if we focus on the Prana, enriching and strengthening it—its power has the capacity to override disease. We can enhance our Prana by enhancing our breath. Paying attention to our breath, learning how to deepen the breath, and practicing breathing exercises will magnify our Prana, or life force.

Pause, now and take three deep breaths. Feel that? That's your life-force coursing through your veins and revitalizing your cells. Spending time in nature will intensify your Prana. Nature is a symphony of life force. Trees, grass, rivers, streams, sunlight, seas, mountains, soil and flowers are included in the planet's generous offering of Prana. Get your hands dirty in the garden, bring plants into your environment, and walk in nature. At some point in your life you have likely been hiking, swimming in the ocean, or on a road trip with your windows down and the wind blowing while taking in the awe inspiring beautiful scenery. Did you feel alive? Did you feel like a puppy with it's head out the windows? So untroubled you surely had stars glistening in your joyful eyes. Of course. That's because when we immerse ourselves in the cosmic dance of life force that covers and sustains this planet, we feel better. Nature is Prana. Part of the reason you feel so great after your yoga practice is because the quality and quantity of Prana within you has been inflated. Prana also comes in Pranic rich foods, like bright and fresh fruits, vegetables, seeds, honey, ghee and whole grains. These whole foods came from the goodness of nature. They are generously packed with the viability of nature. They are robust in all things life force—from anti-oxidants, vitamins, minerals, flavonoids, colors, and textures, to tastes. Because these plants were once basking, flourishing, and blossoming in the most essential and purist of ways they will assist you in doing the same. Indulge in these guiltless pleasures. Breath, nature and whole foods should be some of your dearest companions. Prana is readily accessible, free and delectable medicine.

"The body is a printout of our experiences."

—Deepak Chopra

Grasping the Mind-Body Connection. As a holistic form of medicine, Ayurveda embraces the mind, body, soul, and interconnection of the three. There are three eras of medicine. The first era views the body as a machine; a collection of mechanical pieces and parts. This where we look at specific systems as separates. The nervous system being on functioning system apart from the reproductive system for instances. Era one medicine is concerned with particular organs and their particular functions. Era one medicine does not embrace the perspective that the body is a unified field, where everything can effect everything else. The current model of "specialist" is grounded in era one medicine. You entrust specific zones of your body with specific doctors who are specialist in that zone. This is like looking at a quilt as separate patches of fabric.The second era of medicine recognizes the physiological aspect of the self. This is where the acknowledgment of the placebo effect and physiatrics come into play. Era two understands that there is a mental and emotional component to ones wellbeing, however the mental and emotional bodies are not necessarily treated as integrated aspects of the whole. This is kind of like looking at quilt and since the quilt is more than just patches of fabric. Surely the quilt had a designer and seamstress who created it. Someone probably attributes sentimental value to the quilt, but we do not understand how the patches, designer, maker and owner play together. The third era of medicine appreciates the intrinsic connection between the mind, body, and soul. Ayurveda honors that we are more than the some total of our parts. Everything we think, see, say and do plays a role in the fabric of who we are. We are an intricate tapestry of form, thought, beliefs, ideals and the divine.

On some level, we all understand that our feelings and the way we think effect our bodies. That's why we use phrases like, "Ew, he makes me sick," "That gives me chills," "I have to trust my gut," and "She gives me butterflies." We realize our feelings translate into bodily responses, and bodily responses are reflective of our feelings. There's no single, definitive translation as to how our feelings express themselves in the physical form, but the more I connect with people the more patterns I begin to see. For every psychological experience there is a corresponding physiological experience. For example, if we relentlessly hold on to things emotionally or cling mentally, the body holds and clings too. This can manifest in the holding of the bowels, leading to constipation or the holding of weight—leading to obesity. Have you heard the expression, "Emotionally constipated?" The expression is a play on truth. If we chronically feel life is "hard," our tissues get hard. This leads to uncomfortable musculoskeletal stiffness, and a rigid mind that atrophies in its ability to be pliable in attitudinal or behavioral conditioning. If we're constantly thinking, anxious and worried—our faces wear the lines of our concerns. Our brows become pinched, and sleep becomes disrupted as the waves of spectrums and fear dance behind our foreheads. If we are angry or deceitful, our feelings can eat away at us creating heated skin issues, and hot digestive irritations. The idea of someone being "so uptight," is illustrated in the body as raised and tense shoulders, and tightness in the furrow of the brow. The body is constantly adjusting and adapting to mimic our feelings, attitudes and behaviors. Becoming aware of our thoughts is increasingly important in becoming the director of our lives. It is difficult or near impossible to observe and evaluate thoughts while dancing with the incessant flow of more thoughts. That is why according to *The Law of Attraction,* we simultaneously have thoughts AND feelings. According to this principle, anytime we have an adverse feeling, that is a signal that we need to become aware of our current thought, and adjust the thought to create a feeling we desire. The next time you have an undesirable feeling, immediately pause and ask yourself, "What was that thought?" The quicker we recognize the thought, the easier it is re-route the thought before the insidious feeling becomes chronic or deeply imbedded. It is not necessary to try to watch and catch every thought and feeling. I think that may personally drive me nuts, but when I notice an undesirable feeling reappear several times, I find it worthwhile to see where it is coming from.

There is an open channel of communication between the body, mind and soul. The network of communication between the body, mind and soul is interlaced, so everything effects everything. Eastern Medicine (both Ayurveda and Traditional Chinese Medicine) align particular organs with specific emotional counterparts. The stories of our lives live in our in our cells and tissues. Classical texts explain that the lungs hold grief, the liver governs anger, the kidneys correlate with fear, the large intestine aligns with anxiety, and the heart manufactures love and forgiveness. Emotions create protein-like molecules called neuropeptides that serve as mediators of mental activity as they spread throughout the body. The web between the body, mind and soul is nuanced and intertwined.

Ayurveda connects the Doshas to specific emotions and capacities as well… When Vata is balanced, there is a surge of imagination, intuition, spontaneity and adaptability. Because of this emotional make up—Vatas have an aptitude for art, dance, spirituality and teaching. Vatas should harness their natural creative flare and trust their strong instinct. When Vata is out of balance, fear, anxiety, insecurity, and forgetfulness are more present. The seat, or home base of Vata is in the colon. Vata types are prone to anxiety, therefore they are also prone to constipation. While Vatas are flexible and adaptable they should take special care in creating structure and bolstering their talents with a supportive routines as to stay grounded, and free from anxiety.

When Pitta is in balance, she is ambitious, charismatic and willful. Thanks to Pitta's emotional characteristics, Pittas have a proficiency for productivity and leadership. Pittas should harness their natural drive and funnel it into projects and services they find meaningful. When Pitta is out of balance, there is criticism, anger, irritability and pride. The main site of Pitta Dosha in the body is in the small intestine. When too much heat congregates in this area a person will feel a heat based emotional and physical impact. Pittas should be mindful to schedule rest and play into their determined and orderly schedules. Pittas will find that taking time to chill-out paradoxically helps them reach their goals.

When Kapha is in balance, she is loyal, patient, kind and nurturing. People with predominately Kapha traits have a natural capacity for cooking, healing, and offering support for others— whether that's through hospitality, medicine or executive assistance. It is important for a Kapha that they are not so committed to helping others that they neglect themselves. They should introduce an equally strong sense of support and care into their personal development.

When Kapha is out of balance, the person can become complacent, greedy, lazy and depressed. The seat of Kapha is in the stomach and lung area, this is why Kaphas can suffer from heaviness after eating along with respiratory issues. It is imperative that Kaphas fuse movement and lightness into their daily life, so they do not become heavy and stagnant physically or emotionally. We can access the body through the mind, and the mind through the body. The lines of communication run both ways.

We cannot sever the ties of the interdependent relationship of mind and body. We can assimilate this awareness into our lives, and use it as medicine. Ayurveda describes disease as the blockage of awareness. With awareness, we can restore balance.

In watching clients, I see shared experiences that affirm that getting the ball rolling in the right direction clears the path for incremental growth. Once one feels the progress, the positive feeling of progress leads to monumental momentum. The body and the mind correct in tandem with one another.

> **Practice:** *In times of anxiety, stress or a consuming emotion—take pause. Close your eyes and gently scan your body. Locate the physical location of the emotion. How is it expressing itself in the body? Simply step back and breathe into it. You can infuse your breath with a white light that purifies and nourishes that space. You can attach a mantra or affirmation to the breath. Allow the breath, attention, and intention to target that specific area. Sometimes when I get stressed I can feel the area of around my heart tighten and my brows become tense. I softly close my eyes, scan my face, and encourage my brows to relax. I breathe into my heart and say to myself, "I feel my face relax. I feel my heart relax. I am calm. I am relaxed." After a few moments of this, I feel my nervous system return to neutral. My face softens, my chest loosens up, and I feel better. Adopting this technique will be instantly beneficial for your long term health.*

Catharsis [ke THarses] noun.

> *(1) The purging or release of emotional tensions, esp. through kinds of art and music.*

How to Balance the Doshas: Highlights and Tips:

Vata types are like the wind. They are quick, subtle, unpredictable, enthusiastic, and creative beings. Vata types are always moving. Their bodies are active. Make them sit still and they will talk. Make them be quiet and their minds will dash and scurry with thoughts. Sound familiar? If you or someone in your family is a Vata you have probably noticed a trail of erratic patterns. Vatas can be picky eaters. Sometimes they run to the table starving, other times they'll forget to eat all day. They may seem very cheerful and social one minute, and insecure and withdrawn the next. Vatas tend to be irregular with digestion, sleep and energy. So what to do?

Ground a Vata. Reduce stimulation. Excess sensory input like TV, computer games, bright lights and quick-tempo music irritate Vata. Reduce light, dry, cold and rough foods. Living on snacks of salads and crackers will send Vata through the roof. Give them structure. It is hard to tame the wind, but routine helps.

The qualities of Vata are mobile, quick, light, cold, dry and rough (as mentioned, this also applies to skin, hair and nails).

Tips to Balance Vata:

1. Consume warm and moist food such as hot cereal, soups, and root vegetables.
2. Establish a routine, create a schedule for meals, activities and sleep.
3. Drink ginger tea to improve digestion (Vatas are prone to gas and bloating-try Detox & Replenish Tea by Wellblends)
4. Use ghee and coconut oil for cooking to keep the joints moist and bowels moving

5. Unplug at night. Read or listen to calming music. (Vatas are likely to have light sleep or even insomnia), taking time to unwind, while removing excess stimulus will help.

6. Rub sesame oil on the body before showering. Daily oil massage will calm the nervous system and moisturize the body from the outside in.

7. Limit caffeine. Vatas are programmed to be hyper stimulated. Stimulants can make them anxious, worried, hyper and unfocused.

8. Within a schedule, give Vatas time and space to express their bodies and creativity. A dance or writing class might be a good avenue for a Vata type. Whether it's in an orchestrated setting or at home, Vatas need a creative outlet.

9. Give time for rest. A busy, hurried, over scheduled lifestyle will exacerbate Vata imbalances.

10. Be gentle with a Vata. Vatas will run away or shut down if you're aggressive. We all want to feel good.

Apply these guidelines to a Vata constitution or Vata imbalance. For a Vata type, the reinforcements of regularity and tranquility are indispensable. The emphasis for people with Vata constitutions and Vata imbalances should be on grounding. The keywords for Vata are Slow and Warm.

PAUSE FOR AFFIRMATION

"I am taking my time. I am expressing myself from a place of being rooted and grounded."

Pittas are like fire. Pittas are doers. They are task, goal, and success oriented. These types love planning, organizing, managing and leading. Pittas have a ravenous appetite for food and knowledge. With strong appetites, it's wise to keep a Pitta well fed to dodge irritability, frustration and anger. Pittas may love spicy food, but this should be avoided because it feeds the hot and acidic qualities in the body, (inflammation, excess bile, loose stools and skin issues are not uncommon for a Pitta type). Pittas typically thrive off school, work and competition. It's useful to remind a Pitta that everything doesn't have to be done now, by themselves, or perfectly. Pittas occasionally need to be doused in refreshing water to cool their fierce approach to life. Heating substances like coffee, red meat, alcohol and citrus should be limited. Too much exposure to sun and heat should be minimized.

The qualities of Pitta are light, hot, sharp, spreading, penetrating and oily (this also applies to hair and skin)

Tips to Balance Pitta:

1. Avoid solar colors like red, orange, and bright yellow. Wear clothes, drive cars, and paint rooms blue, green and taupe. (Watery and earthy colors simmer Pitta Dosha)

2. Reduce heating foods are drinks like coffee, chocolate, hard liquor, chili peppers, tomatoes, garlic and onions, to name a few.

3. Avoid eating while conducting business.
   Leave the workspace for meals.

4. Enjoy water sports like kayaking,
   paddle boarding, and swimming.

5. Rub coconut on the body before bed.
   This is cooling and calming.

6. Snack on watermelon, cucumbers and
   coconuts. This will keep 'hanrgy' at bay.

7. Remind Pittas to be patient with others. Not everyone
   is as determined and willful, but that doesn't mean
   they are not providing a valuable contribution.

8. Drink chamomile tea before bed.
   Again, cooling and calming.

9. Spritz rose water on the face and chest.
   It's sweet and refreshing to a Pitta.

10. When applying strategies to balance Pitta,
    keep it playful. Pittas are already serious about
    becoming better. Keep it light and joyful!

The emphasis for people with Pitta constitution or Pitta imbalances should be on Cooling. Keywords for Pitta types are Sweet and Relaxed.

PAUSE OF AFFIRMATION

"I am accomplishing my goals in a relaxed manner."

Kaphas are the contented chill types. Kaphas are snuggly and mellow. These types tend to be sentimental and loyal. Kaphas tend to hold onto things: weight, memorabilia, good friends, concert tickets from 1992, and so on. If you know a hoarder, it's likely you know a Kapha. But wow, Kaphas are sweet! Everyone loves a Kapha. They have a nurturing disposition that lends itself to exceptional care-taking. Kaphas enjoy sugar and dairy but they should shy away from such foods because they are heavy and mucus building. Kaphas tend to suffer from allergies, a milky metabolism, and respiratory issues—so it's best to keep their food light and heating. For example a broth based bean chili is ideal. Too many dreary days in a row can send Kaphas into couch potato mode, so keep Kaphas moving and catching rays as often as possible.

The qualities of Kapha are cold, heavy, dull, slimy, sticky, dense and slow. Add in the opposites to secure balance. Warm, light and quick activities and food options best serve Kapha types.

Tips to Balance Kapha:

1. Drink ginger/cinnamon/clove tea to amp up circulation and metabolism. (Kaphas tend to have sluggish digestive capacities and stagnant circulation.)

2. Give a Kapha variety. These people are creatures of habit and comfort. Shake things up a bit with curveballs and spontaneity.

3. Try to eat a bigger lunch and lighter dinner. Kaphas will wake up lazy or congested if they eat too much or too late.

4. Let them cuddle, pet and adore. Kaphas love to cuddle, pet and adore.

5. Keep Kapha stimulated with movement, spices and bright neon colors.

6. Grab a loofah brush and enjoy a brisk dry rub to shake off heaviness, break up adipose tissue, surge circulation and jazz up the nervous system. (Kaphas are the exact opposite of Vatas in this regard.)

7. Wake up early! Kaphas like sleeping-in, but waking up with the sun will burn away any potential malaise.

8. Play sports. Kaphas are strong and have mighty endurance. Take advantage of it.

9. Keep eucalyptus essential oil in your car or at your desk. Rub a few drops in your palm and inhale. This will lift your energy and open your sinuses.

10. Kaphas require a bit of reminding, external motivation, and maybe a little push to create change. Be respectful, but also firm while implementing these Kapha balancing suggestions.

The emphasis for people with Kapha constitutions and Kapha imbalances is Lightness. The keywords for Kapha are Movement and Heat.

PAUSE OF AFFIRMATION

"I am light and energetic."

CHAPTER FOUR

Rhythms and Ease

The Dalai Lama, when asked what surprised him most about humanity—he answered, "Man, because he sacrifices his health in order to make money. Then he sacrifices his money to recuperate his health. And then he is so anxious about the future that he does not enjoy the present, the result being that he does not live in the present or the future -he lives as if he is never going to die, and then he dies having never really lived."

EVERYTHING ON EARTH Runs on Rhythm: Moon cycles, the tides, the seasons, the development from conception through old age, and our heart beat all synchronize to a specific rhythm. Ayurveda teaches us to sync our lives with the master rhythm—these are the universal tempos. We have come to a collective agreement in our relationship with time. We agree there are sixty-seconds in a minute, sixty minutes in an hour, twenty-four hours in a day, seven days in a week, and twelve months in a year. We all feel pretty confident that the sun will rise in the morning and set at night (unless you live in Alaska, Iceland or the like, but even there you've come to accept the rhythms of a sunlit summer and dark winter). These are all functions of the master rhythm. Recognizing stability and patterns regarding time helps us organize and make the most of each moment. In a quick moving world with a clamorous amount of options, and much to do, a sustainable rhythm will carry you through.

> *"Rhythm is something you either have or you don't, But when you have it, you have it all over."*
>
> **—Elvis Presley**

Nature is in harmony with rhythms and time. Nature is calibrated by a brilliant universal clock. Animals instinctually and habitually function in accordance to this rhythm of time. For most of human existence, we were connected to these rhythms as well. We got up with the sun, and went to sleep with the moon. But with the advent of the lightbulb and ensuing modern devices, we can carry on with business and pleasure 24-7. I love technology as much as the next person, but technology and modern conveniences have caused us to become desensitized to the master rhythm.

How often do we fight the clock? How often do we ignore the rhythmic messages of the body? The mentality of too much to do, in too little time can drive us to attempt to mask the legitimate need to rest with copious amounts of caffeine and stimulants. When we get out of sync, we come supercharged at inappropriate times . We fall into the corrosive habit of trying to compensate through sedatives, alcohol, or dulling distractions. Unreliable daily routines, stimulants, and sedatives all alter our relationship with the master rhythm. The master rhythm provides a template as to when it is to best perform certain activities. We are nature. Nature doesn't fight itself. Vata, Pitta and Kapha govern various times of day in accordance to the clock. These determined blocks of day lend themselves to specific energies and functions. When we match our rhythm to the master rhythm, we are able to accentuate our capabilities by gaining the support of the broader spectrum of energies

> *"I could be a morning person… If morning happened around noon."*
>
> **— An Unknown Kapha**

The Master Clock…Here's how it works: According to ancient Ayurvedic texts 2-6am is Vata time of day. Vata is light and quick, so your sleep may be disturbed at this time. How many of us wake up around 3am? It's very common. According to Ayurveda, during Vata times of day the veil between the earthly realm and the cosmic realm is at its thinnest. That is way you may wake up with a burst of energy, inspiration or wellspring of creativity. This is the time of day when we hear the whispers of the stars. Wayne Dyer, my favorite author and teacher, often woke up at 3:13am and wrote many of his books in those peak twilight hours. The beautiful poet, Rumi said, "The breeze at dawn has secrets to tell you. Don't go back to sleep. You must ask for what you really want. Don't go back to sleep. People are going back and forth across doorsill where the two worlds touch, the door is round and open. Do not go back to sleep!" I understand this may seem impractical if you have to wake up early to go to work, and you'd feel braindead or like a zombie if you were to follow Rumi's advice of staying up at 3am, but the theory still stands. According to Ayurveda, if you wake up at 3am it's best to express this light and fast energy through creativity or reflection. Journal or meditate. To calm Vata at this time, you can rub sesame oil on the soles of your feet, spritz your pillow with lavender, or sip on chamomile tea or Golden Milk to go back to bed for a few hours. Should you snooze through the 3am hour, good for you, however it is still best to rise during the Vata time of day. Given you went to bed at a reasonable hour, waking up before 6am will illuminate your cells with the sprightly energy of Vata, infusing your day with liveliness. Ayurveda states that 6-10am is Kapha time of day. The morning Kapha hours can be used to capitalize on Kapha's strength and endurance. This is the best time for exercise or manual labor like cutting the grass. You can use Kapha's loyal endurance to plough through to-do lists, chores and errands during this time. Sleeping into the peak Kapha hours such as 8-9am will layer you with a blanket of Kapha energy for the entire all day. This energy is heavy and slow. Heavy and slow may be perfect for a Sunday, but less than ideal when you have a busy day ahead. Have you ever noticed how sleeping too long actually makes you feel more tired? That is because sleep saturates you with heavy, slow and stable qualities. Too much of anything can create an imbalance…even sleep. 10am-2pm is Pitta time of day. Pitta gives fire and ambition. Maximize Pitta's ability to transform by eating your biggest meal at this time. This is when both the sun and the gut are at their apex. Take advantage of it. Eat your biggest meal here. Tasks that employ your ambition, passion and charisma should be done during the Pitta hours. Because Pitta is sharp, this is the best time to enroll your cognitive functions. Put your thinking cap on, mentally demanding work and study sessions should be placed here. Then the clock circles back around… 2-6pm, Here Vata energy is back in full swing. Due to the volatile nature of Vata, you may notice your energy peaks and dips during these hours. You have likely felt that 3pm dip and then a second wind around 5pm. It is best to ground Vata by connecting with nature—taking a slow and steady mindful walk, or taking a few conscious breaths during these hours will help stabilize your swings. Creativity and movement are heightened at this time of day. Draw, dance, write and create.

> *"I try to manage my day by my circadian rhythms because creativity is such an elusive thing, and I could easily just stomp over it doing administrative stuff."*
>
> **—Scott Adams (cartoonist)**

6-10pm, Here the heavy and slow qualities of Kapha return. This is nature's way of hinting we should wind-down. Eat a light dinner, take a slow stroll and relax. It is advisable to unplug during the latter hours of this phase. Unplug from electronics and gadgets by 9pm or 10pm. Electronic devices emit blue waves. These high frequency lights disturb our pineal gland, and interfere with our natural ability to create the hormone melatonin, which helps regulate our wake/sleep cycles. This is the best time to go to bed. This bracket of time lends itself to tranquility and peaceful rest. 10pm-2am, Pitta is back. If you stay up past 10:30pm or 11pm you may notice a second wind. A second burner clicks on. You can become hungry and ambitious all over again. Go to bed before peak Pitta hours to avoid raiding the kitchen, or writing a dissertation at midnight. We should not be burning energy during this bracket of time because this energy is needed for the body to restore and repair while we rest. Each organ has a specific time in which it repairs, for example the stomach regenerates at midnight, and the liver detoxes at 2am. If we are up during these pivotal hours, we miss out on a chance to internally restore.

"I'm envious of people who can sleep as long as they want. I have the circadian rhythm of a farmer."

—Moby

PAUSE FOR AFFIRMATION

"I am in alignment with the natural harmony of life."

A Stress Free Lifestyle Please: Trying to have more, do more, and be more are ingredients for unnecessary stress. The unrelenting mentality of 'more' as become the cultural epidemic of our time. Stress constricts and blocks our energy. Studies show 75% of modern illnesses are rooted in stress. Stress weakens our immunity, impairs our capacity to digest thoroughly, throws our hormones out of whack, diminishes our sleep, and hinders our ability to think clearly, and react peacefully. Did you know more heart attacks occur on Monday morning than only other day of the week? The anticipation of stressful events is enough to trigger an outpour of stress hormones like adrenaline and cortisol that overwhelms the body. It's no secret that stress contributes to a host of undesirable imbalances. Luckily for us, reducing stress is as enjoyable as it is essential.

"You retain your health only so long as you are willing to forgive stresses, shrug off adversity and adapt to new situations. Resisting the change always impedes the workings of your immunity."

—Robert E. Svoboda

Reducing stress may be as simple as swapping the chatter on the radio for an inspirational CD, an enlightening podcast, or ambient sounds. Prioritizing your to-dos and deleting the ones that at second look seem inconsequential. Blocking time in your schedule to do, dare I say it? Nothing. Read or take a stroll instead of cramming in more tasks. Reduce how much time you on social media; Facebook, twitter and the like. These outlets can easily consume precious time without adding core value. Staring at screens and gadget depletes our precious Prana reserves. Limit screen time. Delegate. Devi up chores so everyone in the house contributes equally. Structure your day effectively regarding routes and locations of meeting and errands to eliminate extra time in traffic. Even good stressors such as social events, parties and planning can tax the nervous system. If our schedules are constantly jam packed we are left without ample time and space to experience the good taste of relaxation.

Recently, after a long week I woke up on a Saturday morning excited to go to Disney with my family. But when I go there something unexpected and strange happened. I immediately became overwhelmed and extraordinarily sensitive to the incessant noise and stimulation. I love my family more than words can express, but I suddenly needed to leave. I said goodbye and got an uber home. The uber driver said, "It's unusual for me to pick someone up from Disney so early in the day." I briefly told him how I became overwhelmed by the hustle and bustle of the crowds, and felt I needed to remove myself from that environment. When he dropped me off he said, "I hope you enjoy spending the rest of the day you want, verses the way other people want." He was right. I did. I went home showered, gave myself a coconut oil massage, applied a beauty mask, and spent the evening editing the pages you're reading now. I initially felt a bit unsettled about not spending time with my family, but I realize that honoring what you need pays dividends to the people you love in the long run.

While implementing the entire plethora of ideas on how to reduce stress and mitigate overwhelming commitments may not be within your immediate grasp, you can certainly incorporate the tools that resonate with you in our own way, in your own time. We are all working within a perimeter of limitations and opportunities. We have to customize our strategies to fit our unique realities. A steadfast mission to reduce stress should not incite stress. Toy around with some of these suggestions, consider subscribing to the idiom, "Less is more."

> *"The key is not to prioritize what's on your schedule. The key is to schedule your priorities."*
>
> **—Steven Covey**

There are sneaky stressors too. Stressors like violent images, crude words, startling or loud noises and harsh smells. These stressors impact our nervous system, digestion, and emotional atmosphere. As a function of Pitta, and our ability to metabolize and transform—all of our impressions and experiences are digested, absorbed and assimilated into the fabric of who we are. On a moment to moment basis, every impression and experience can either add stress or bring peace. Be mindful of the music you listen to, TV shows and movies your watch, surroundings you plant yourself in, and even the conversations you entertain. Everything has an energy—every word, color, sound, impulse, and action will somehow translate into your nervous system, thereby affecting the organs of the body. This impressions are not contained to the organs, they spill into the spirit and touch the soul. Try to create, and consume peaceful impressions as much as possible.

"Dear Stress,… Let's break up."

—Anonymous

Busy-oholics: Author Brene Brown said, "If we had meetings for busy-oholics, we would fill stadiums." It is true. We are creatures equipped with intelligent and equally delicate biorhythms. Our culture of 24-7 productivity and stimulation discombobulates our biorhythms resulting in stress, anxiety, frustration, disturbed sleep, and a perpetual inclination to do more. As a culture, we have become addicted to and intoxicated by a constant need to do something, see something, be something…the proverbial list goes on. Ceaseless stimulation defies the natural law that asks us to rest and unplug. Michael Jefferys said, "Every second you spend looking for something outside yourself is another second you spend away from your true nature." I've personally caught myself spending too much time on social media. I'll check Facebook and Instagram in the morning, catch myself looking at it again at a stop light, occasionally again in-between appointments, and yet again before bed. Studies show the average American checks social media seventeen times a day. The allure for entertainment and distraction are worrisome.

Brown says of busy-oholics, we tend to believe, "If we stay busy enough the truth of our lives won't catch up with us." When I initially heard that I winced a little. I know for me, that a sign I absorbed a truth that pierced a very real place in my life. Social media can be a wonderful platform for sharing, connecting, learning, and finding inspiration. However, it can also be a vice or distraction, interfering with our ability to nourish what we are actually hungry for. Researchers now use the term "hyper-communication". A large amount of communication is not mutual exclusive to effective or satisfying communication. Communicating is different from connecting. When it comes to seeking connection, quantity is better than quantity. I've come to realize, when i'm feeling lonely a walk with a friend nourishes me more than, "likes" or, "comments" on social media. I practice witnessing myself on days where I'm reaching for icons, browsers and apps. I pause and ask myself, "What do I need right now?" The answer is not typically immediate available, but the questions provokes the ensuing thought…"I deserve what I actually need". And that is enough to make me feel better. To be in alignment with our True Nature and universal nature, we have to slow down. We must give ourselves permission to do less, and take refuge in the still, quiet spaces between the doing. We are worthy and deserving. We are safe to unplug. Breathing, meditation, yoga, time in nature, self-care, and a good nights sleep are paramount in nurturing a stress free lifestyle. Ayurveda and yoga refer to our need and ability to reduce stimulation as Pratyahara, or control of the senses. Pratayahara suggests that we develop a mastery of external influences by withdrawing from our senses. I recently discovered sensory deprivation tanks. They are essentially huge pods filled with a shallow depth of magnesium rich salt water. You lie in the pod, close the hatch and rest in complete silence and darkness. An hour or so later, you lift the lid of the pod and enter back into the world that requires the use of your senses. I find it intriguing and therapeutic. I wouldn't recommend it for those who are claustrophobic, but otherwise, it offers an effortless outlet for practicing Pratayahara.

Practice: *It's challenging to make improvements without knowing what exactly needs to be improved upon. That would be like a contractor trying to renovate a kitchen without a blue print of the kitchen. I find it helpful to grasp what i'm dealing with, and elevating my awareness by making a list or diagram of my schedule, activities, tasks, commutes and hobbies. If you want to try this, be specific. Place smiley faces next to activities that are stress free. Draw frown faces next to stressful activities. You can prioritize your list by place numbers near the tasks. A ten means it's of the utmost importance, a zero signifies that it's inconsequential. You'll get a visual representation of what you are currently working with. From there, you can play around with modifying your current lifestyle and schedule in a way that will reduce your stress.*

Poem…

I'm tired of dates.

Of being ruled by a clock,

Steered by an agenda,

And governed by a tightly packed schedule.

I'm tired of having to say yes,

And no.

Of needing to please

Others

And myself.

Of giving giving and giving

And needing

Oh so many needs.

I'm tired of not being there for people I love.

Weary by the space that business creates between those to whom I was once close

And now

We're distant.

My remedy I suppose is being energized by time

A time that truly does not exist.

It's a moment that lapses into another moment

And another.

Moments strung together like a pearl laced to a pearl, laced to a pearl.

A necklace of life.

I'm rejuvenated by the knowing that everything I "have" to do is truly not an obligation, but a privilege.

I don't "have" to do anything

I get to do

And that's an honor.

And to the people I love,

Know that I am trying

And you are trying.

And distance may nudge between us,

But the space between us is not mine.

It's not yours.

The space is ours. We share it. And I'll meet you there.

And to Self, the girl who is thinking these thoughts and wearing these worries.

You are loved.

And you are doing well.

You may disappoint others and be disappointed yourself,

But darling, your existence is complete.

You are here to be the bringer of joy.

You are here to travel through life to completion.

Let yourself fall in love. Let your heart break. Let yourself be dedicated, playful, and brave. Show your scars. Undress from your armor. Cry. When the sun drops, let your hair down and be wild. Sleep hard. And when the sun rises, be renewed. You are here to love and be loved.

My love, don't let expectations rob you of that.

CHAPTER FIVE

Breathe and Meditation

"Meditation: because some questions can not be answered by Google."

—Anonymous

BREATHE... OXYGEN IS ONE of the most vital healing resources in existence. Take a deep breath—become aware and calm, boost your immunity, and heal. Breathing practices have special Sanskrit name called, Pranayama. Pranayama means, breath control. You will recall that the word Prana means life force or vitality. Remember that one of the best ways to enhance your health is to invite in more Prana. We receive Prana through multiple sources, sunlight and nature, wholesome food (plants) and oxygen…breath! Allow me to guide you through several breathing practices. The first is called three part breath. It is short, sweet, and immediately calming. Have you ever watched a baby sleep? They peacefully breathe into their bellies. Over the years, the cumulative effects of stress cause our breath to rise from the relaxed zone of the belly into the caged area of the chest. This technique will reestablish your intrinsic connection to untroubled belly breathing. Three part breath is effective because it shifts you into to the parasympathetic nervous system. This system is responsible for a slowing the heart rate and relaxing smooth muscles. You can lie down or sit up tall. The most important part is that you're comfortable. You can practice this breathing pattern for as little as three cycles, (rounds) or up to five or ten minutes. There's no harm in going longer, but you'll probably find five to ten minutes to be plenty.

Three Part Breath (Dirga Pranayama)

To begin:

» Place your right hand over your heart and your left hand over your belly.

» Feel the natural rise and fall of the belly and chest as you breath.

» Allow the air to enter and exit at its own will.

» Just observe the breath for a few cycles.

» Once you've familiarized yourself with the nature of your breath, exhale completely.

» Breathing through the nose, inhale into the belly, and pause. (You'll feel air fill your belly like a balloon being inflated.)

» Now sip in more air and fill the whole chest, and hold. (You'll feel your side ribs flare open like fish gills.)

» At the top of the breath, increase your lung capacity by gently sipping in a little more air, and retain.

- » Before you reach the point of discomfort, exhale through the mouth.
- » Repeat this cycle as many times as you'd like.

Alternate Nostril Breathing (Nadi Shodhan Pranayama) You will need to sit up tall for this one. You can sit on the floor if that's comfortable for you, or you can sit in a chair and plant your feet firmly on the ground. The important part is that your spine is straight because the spine is the storehouse for the central nervous system, and the main channel for the energy that runs up and down the body. This called the "Sushumna Nadi", or Central Channel. A Nadi is a channel of energy that creates a tube or pathway for energy to flow. There are 72,000 Nadis in the body. The three most significant Nadis or channels are the Central (Sushumna), The channel on the righthand side, that correlates with masculine energy, (Pingala), and the channel on the left, that correlates with feminine energy, (Ida). The seven Chakras or wheels, sometimes called reservoirs of energy, run up the Central Channel.The channels that run on the right (Pingala) and left (Ida) sides of the spine weave up the central channel like a serpentine. We would need a whole book to explore this concept in depth, but for the sake of background information—there are thousands of pathways, three main channels and seven reservoirs of energy. Think of the channels,(Nadis) as rivers and the reservoirs, (Chakras) as springs. We want our rivers to flow, and our springs to bubble. For all intents and purposes, that is all we need to know here.

Alternate nostril breathing clears the channels, and harmonizes the right/masculine, and left/feminine sides of the mind-body. It balances both hemispheres of the brain. While the whole brain contributes to the entirety of the way we operate, the left hemisphere of the brain dominates logic and pragmatic thinking, while the right hemisphere governs creativity and intuition. This breath helps us synchronize communication between the two sides of the brain. Alternate nostril breathing also balances the Yin (passive), and Yang (active) aspects of the self, and fosters an equilibrium in feminine and masculine aspects of the self, thereby helping to balance hormone regulation . We all have Yin and Yang, passive and active, aspects irrespective of our gender, or tendencies. Our most dominate feminine hormones are estrogen and progesterone, while the driving masculine hormones are testosterone and cortisol. No matter what sex we are, these hormones and corresponding chemicals course through our veins. How amazing is it that a breathing practice can help us achieve balance in both the body and mind? The reason this works is because the nasal canal is the pathway to consciousness. The breath enters and exits through the nose, and spirals up and down the spine like a loose braid or a serpentine snake. To get a visual, you can picture the double helix of the DNA. This breathing exercise essentially cleanses the channels, while guiding us back balance without trying. It happens naturally.

Alternate Nostril Breathing *(This exercise will prove itself tricky if you're suffering from a cold or severe congestion. Select a different breathing technique until your nasal passage way clears.)*

To Begin:

» Sit up tall.

» Lengthen your spine.

» Allow your shoulders to drop down away from the ears. Relax.

- » Allow your chin to run level with the ground, (do not tilt your chin up).
- » With your left hand, bring your index finger and thumb together to touch (this will create a little Mudra or seal).
- » Rest that hand on your left knee, or in your lap.
- » With your right hand, invite your pointer finger and middle finger to rest at the space between your eyebrows.
- » Now your thumb and ring finger are available and ready for use. You'll be using your right hand only for this practice.You will be breathing through the nose the entire time, (your mouth will remain closed).
- » Exhale.
- » With your right thumb, plug your right nostril and inhale through the left.
- » With your right ring finger, plug you left nostril and exhale through the right nostril.
- » Stay on the same side. With your ring finger, plug the left nostril and inhale through the right nostril.
- » Alternate sides.
- » With your thumb, plug the right nostril, and inhale through the left.
- » With the ring finger, plug the left nostril and exhale through the right.
- » Keep using your fingers in the same manner.
- » Inhale through the right, exhale through the left.

- » Inhale through the left, exhale through the right.
- » Continue with this pattern for 2-10 minutes. The duration of time is flexible. Practice the technique until you feel the balancing effects. This could happen in two minutes or twenty minutes. It would be very hard to overdose on breath, so don't feel restricted to a specific length of time.

"Everything is unfolding perfectly, and as you relax and find ease in your attitude of trust knowing that wellbeing is yourself birthright amazing things will happen. Things like you have no seen before."

—Abraham

Relaxation Breath

To Begin:

- » Exhale completely.
- » Breathing through the nose, inhale for four counts, (seconds), and pause.
- » Retain the breath for six counts, (seconds).
- » Slowly exhale through the nose for seven counts, (seconds)

Repeat this pattern 3-5 times or for several minutes. You will experience a sense of inner tranquility.

SO HUM

The next breathing exercise is as powerful as it is uncomplicated. This is called "SO HUM". The meaning of SO HUM is I AM. SO HUM, or I AM, is the Mantra, or affirmation we have been using throughout the book to strengthen our vibration, frequency, and capacity to attract what we want into our lives. The word Mantra comes from two words, Man (mind) and Tra (training). A Mantra is a valuable tool to help train or reprogram your mind. This technique is a nice way to blend your breathing practice into a meditation practice. This works as a meditation because meditation simply means paying attention on purpose. And guess what, when you are paying attention to your breath or an affirmation, you are paying attention on purpose…therefor you are meditating. Isn't that nice? You can do this practice anywhere. Sitting, lying, standing, at your desk, in an elevator, literally anywhere.

> *"So Hum. I am that I am. The universe exists within me, as much as I exist in the universe."*
>
> **—Unknown**

SO HUM

To Begin:

- Feel comfortable in your surroundings and in your body.
- As you inhale you can think or even say out loud, (if you're in an appropriate/private space) the word, "SO".
- And as you exhale you can think or say out loud the word, "HUM".

Follow this breathing and thinking pattern for as few as 3-5 cycles for as long as 10-20 minutes. You will feel waves of peace sweep over you, calming your mind, and nourishing your soul.

PAUSE FOR AFFIRMATION

"I am giving myself permission to just be."

"Meditation means to record the positive things of your life. When insults, hurts, flattery, and negative things are recorded the brain becomes a trash can. Train your brain to record the authentic."

—Vasant Lad

Meditation makes reality feel lighter…There's an old fable about a hard working man who carried a huge boulder home from work. The boulder was cumbersome, burdensome, and weighed him down. The huge rock represented all of his troubles and woes. The man decided he didn't want to bring his burden into his home to share with his wife and kids, so he made a commitment to leave the gigantic boulder near the front door. He made the assumption he could pick it up again when he left for work in the following morning. He went it. Hugged his kids, kissed his wife, and enjoyed a wonderful evening. To his surprise when he walked out his front door the following morning, he couldn't find his boulder anywhere. He searched high and low. "How did a huge rock just disappear?" He thought. Finally, he looked closely and picked up a tiny pebble. "Is this my boulder? It has become a pebble." He thought. Yes, sometimes problems seem consuming.

However, give them space, shift your perspective, and more often then not—you realize, it was a pebble all along. Meditation helps me realize I often mistake a pebble for a rock. I must admit. I practiced yoga for many years before I became interested in meditation. Initially, I presumed meditation to be an illusory blend of boring, intimidating, and somewhat frightening. I couldn't be more thankful I finally moved past that and made meditation a part of my daily life. The actual act of meditating is relatively anti-climactic, or at least it usually is for me anyway. It is not like there's this glorious light show of radiant colors, concert of angelic string instruments, or parade of epiphanies, and proclamations of wisdom. For me, it is usually just me, sitting there nice and still with a cascade of thoughts, and a few occasional gaps between the thoughts. As the gaps become longer, I feel more and more peaceful. That is it. "That's it?", you ask. "Then why bother?" Fair point. I'll tell you why. Mediation has been proven to spark cellular regeneration. Meditation reduces the effects of aging, memory loss, substance abuse, and stress. Meditation helps us recover gray matter of the brain. It increase focus and cognitive function. Research indicates that it aids in psychiatric disorders, mood swings, and sleep patterns. Meditation calms the nervous system, boosts the immune system, and enhances our ability to come up with creative solutions—while allowing us to harness our energy all day long. Wow! Yes! Meditation really does all of that. Goodness, even if you only accessed a fraction of those benefits, it would be well worth your time. I know for me—meditation has allowed me to feel more composed, trusting and even keeled in my energy and mood patterns. Allow me to continue breaking the ice with this cute story.

There was a woman sitting under a tree and a man walks up and says,

> "What are you doing?"
> The woman responded,"Nothing."
> He said, "You should do something."
> She said, "Why?"
> Clearly they were on different pages.
> He said, "So you can make money."
> She asked, "Why?"
> He said, "So you can buy a house."
> She responded, "Why?"
> He said, "So you can have servants."
> She inquired, "Why?"
> He said, "So you can relax."
> She laughed and thought, "But that's what I'm already doing."

"If you have time to breathe, you have time to meditate."

—Ajahn Chah

I am fortunate to teach yoga, and own a clinic where I have the pleasure of talking with all sorts of people about meditation on a daily basis. The most common comment I hear is, "I'd love to, I just don't have time." I get it. We all have a lot to do, but your meditation practice really doesn't need to consume much of your time. In addition, because meditation will promote your ability to function from a place of deeper clarity. Meditation will actually enable you to be more efficient, thereby saving you time. I was at a conference where a world renowned meditation teacher named David Ji was speaking on the benefits of meditation. David has worked with all sorts of celebrities. He taught meditation to everyone from Bono to Oprah. He made a good point. He said, "Oprah runs a show, magazine, radio station, and philanthropy projects among other things. Perhaps the busiest woman on the planet—she has time to meditate but you.. you don't?" Good point my friend. It wasn't until I started meditation that I realized it seems to glide into my day quite seamlessly, and makes the hours around it much easier to process.

> *"When we meditate we slow ourselves down into stillness and silence so we can finally hear the whisper within our heart."*
>
> **—David Ji**

The world is a candy store when it comes to styles of meditation. There is no need to feel overwhelmed by all of the schools of thought, and options in the field of meditation. You can do no wrong. Whatever lands at your feet, whatever you hear people talking about, whatever you seek out, whatever you resonate with—essentially whatever form you choose, it is correct. For some people, the breathing and Mantra (affirmation) exercise are meditative enough. Other people might explore transcendental meditation, prayer, guided meditations, or Yoga Nidra (guided sleep meditation). Some people like walking meditations, drawing meditations, mindful eating meditations, or even just plain old sitting down with the eyes closed meditation. I'd encourage you to look into Apps on your smartphone. I tend to be archaic my way of thinking and operating in the world. I still use a paper planner, I write my consultation receipts on posit notes, I track my finances in a journal I call my "abundance log," (you can imagine how much my accountant loves that), but one it comes to meditation, paradoxically I embrace technology. There are currently several free Apps that offer wonderful resources and tools for relaxation and meditation, such as Insight Timer and Head Space, to name a few.

> *"We have to develop simplicity. Love is simple. Awareness is simple. Perception is simple. If you think in complications, life will be complicated."*
>
> **—Vasant Lad**

The words Meditation and Medication only have one letter difference. This may be a secret linguistic clue to the magnitude of healing that resides within the practice of meditation. Meditation can sometimes be misunderstood and can have a reputation for being esoteric, because of the preconceived ideas and mysteries that dance around the word. As I mentioned before, meditation just means: paying attention on purpose. Some people feel more comfortable replacing the word meditation with "mindfulness". That works too. The word doesn't really matter. It's the meaning and intention behind the word that counts. I have to be totally honest, meditation freaked me out at first. I was like, "What?! Sit still?! What, don't think?!? What? Don't open my eyes!?!" The whole thing had me befuddled and unsettled. It was not until I realized how simple meditation can be that the fear subsided. First of all, there's no such thing as being, "good" at meditating. So we can go ahead and relieve ourselves of that pressure. Next, we don't need to stop thinking. Hello, it is the nature of the mind to think, that is its primary function. Meditation just allows us to become more conscious of our thoughts. We have between 60,000-80,000 thoughts a day, so please do not feel defeated if you happen to think during meditation. We are cerebral creatures. We all think. The early stage of sitting down for a meditation practice is kind of like the early stage of going to the gym. At first, you may resist it, but just getting there is the hardest part. Once you are there it is can be challenging at first, but as you grow stronger, you gradually increase the length of time to match your degree of comfort. It becomes natural. The ability to rest and do nothing is woven into the programming of our DNA. In time, the experience becomes quite enjoyable. I met with my friend Ashley for a consultation. Ashley was already healthy and in a balanced state. She takes good care of herself, but was seeking advice as to prevent possible woes in the future. One thing she was missing in her life was meditation. After our meeting, she committed to meditating everyday. She relayed to me that she started with a three minute meditation and did well. She then bombed up to five minutes, and was surprised how fast time went. When she did eight minutes, she was shocked that it felt shorter than the three minute meditation. I completely understood what she meant. This happens to me too. I describe it as the, "Dropping in effect." Once the mind runs through the proverbial chatter, it slows down. Once it slows down, we drop into a calmer state where the vibrations are smooth, and seem to exist beyond our ordinary framework of time and space.

Meditating is like strengthening your mindfulness muscles. Meditation benefits us on every level. The effects of meditation untangle knots in our minds, hearts, and bodies. Meditation brings our brainwaves into relaxed states, where creativity flourishes, anxiety disappears, happiness increases, intuition develops, problems become smaller, focus sharpens, awareness expands, and clarity prevails. Physically, meditation lowers blood pressure, boosts the immune system, increases serotonin production, bolsters energy and decreases tension pain such as headaches, ulcers, insomnia and joint stiffness. Perhaps this is why gurus tend to respond to queries with the beloved phrase, "Just meditate." Fitting mediation into your daily routine will require less finagling and finessing, and more prioritizing. There's a saying that you should meditate for twenty minutes a day…unless you do not have time. Then you should meditate for forty minutes. I know, I know, funny Buddha. But really, meditation is not just for monks and mini Buddhas. The accessibility and benefits of meditation are too prevalent and powerful to pass up. Consistent to all improvements, the changes you make should honor your current situation, beliefs and ideals. If you have a resistance, start slow and small. No one is asking you to hurdle out of your comfort zone.

You could designate five minutes in the morning and/or evening to try one of the suggested breathing or meditation exercises. If finding the time and space is tricky, weave your meditation into an existing activity that requires privacy like taking a shower, or using the toilet, (no one said meditating on the pot was illegal). I've meditated in airplanes and public restrooms. I would suggest that you try to meditate in the same space and around the same time each day. Allowing your meditation practice to become habitual relives you from having to make special arrangements for it each day. It becomes as automatic as brushing your teeth. Meditating in the morning is optimal because it sets the tone for the day; this creates space for clarity and inspiration. Meditating in the evening is also advantageous because it can it clear out residual thoughts from the day that may otherwise keep you preoccupied or unsettled. If you choose to meditation once a day, I'd select the morning so that no matter what pops up during the day, the resonance and benefits will accompany you. Similar to the breathing practices, it would be very hard to overdose on meditation. When it comes to developing a practice, two minutes is better than zero minutes.

Meditations per the Doshas: The style of meditation you gravitate towards will be influenced by your Dosha. Obviously, all three Doshas benefit from meditation.

Vatas are the creative, stimulated and energetic types. You should give your mind somewhere to be, or you will either space out into the cosmos, or feel anxious with far too many rapid thoughts. Try calming the nervous system by inhaling through the nose for 4 counts and exhaling through the nose for 8 counts, (You can do this sitting up or lying down.) After that you may try a free guided meditation from your smartphone or youtube, or just try watching your breath. Follow each inhalation and exhalation as though you are utterly fascinated by it. I like to attach my Mantra or affirmation to my breath. For example, "Inhale, I breathe in love. Exhale, I breathe out love. Inhale, I breath in love. Exhale, I breathe out love." When you begin this practice you might just do it for a several minutes a day. If you are looking for a template, I would suggest five to ten minutes morning and night. Vata types benefit the most from stable routines, so create a reliable practice that you do at the same time, in the same place each day. This will help you fortify a sense of stability in your life. Overtime, you may find that you would enjoy expanding the amount of time you spend in quiet stillness. As it begins to feel increasingly natural, the benefits will remind you to come back. Much like going to the gym to acquire a great physique; you don't stop going to the gym once you get buff. No, you continue to go because you know that the muscles will not maintain themselves. The same is true for mindfulness and meditation. It's not like, "Yep, I did. it. Check. Gathered all the benefits, moving on. See ya next year." You always return to the practice. It becomes part of your routine or ritual. Remember, for Vatas specifically—part of the medicine lives in the fact that it is a grounding routine. Pittas are the ambitious, competitive task masters. Pittas will want to be, "good" at meditating. Cool and calm is your motto. You may like to lie down and imagine cool water at the tips of your toes. As you inhale through the nose, draw the breath and water up the body, imagine cool water filling the body like a container. As you exhale through the nose, let the breath and water rinse down the body. Continue filling and emptying the body with this refreshing goodness for several minutes. You will benefit from other styles of guided or seated meditations as well. Explore from a place of playful inquisition, rather than obligation or achievement. I often rave about Insight Timer and guided meditations at workshops. During a workshop, a friend raised his hand to enthusiastically share that he loves Insight Timer because it tracks your stats—sessions, times, and mile marker goals. Pittas love to measure and reach goals. I admit, as a partial Pitta I beamed the first time I saw my stats pop up, "You have meditated X hours in X days." Go on Pittas, track away, but remember the trophy is for your soul; the prize is not on your resume. Kaphas are the grounded mellow types. Meditation comes more naturally to you. You are generally happy to sit and chill, but you might get so comfy you could fall asleep.Try a walking meditation. You can even add a chant, "Loka Samasta Sukhino Bhavantu". This Sanksrit chant means, may all beings everywhere be joyful and free. Kapha types feed off the motivation of other people and thrive in fellowships; Kaphas may consider joining a meditation group or club, whether it be online or in a face to face fellowship. Some of the smart phone Apps have fellowship boards and charts that log your meditation patterns and allow you to connect with people. These kinds of tools will be helpful for you in staying connected, and staying on track. Speaking of fellow ship boards—Cliff, one of my yoga students actually met his long term girlfriend on a meditation app. They were serendipitously frequently meditating at the same time; one day one of them noticed the other, and reached out to connect over their serendipitously aligned meditation routine. Their shared adoration for meditating escalated a close bond. So close, they now travel from Orlando to Asheville to see each other on a monthly basis. The options I mention do not exhaust the list of innumerable ways to meditate. The idea is to slow down, pay attention on purpose, and quiet the chatter so you'll feel calm and centered. I have a client named Liana, who is an extraordinary mother to two miraculous teenage girls, who have both been diagnosed with autism. I introduced Liana to meditation and she immediately wrapped her loving arms around the practice like an old friend her soul had so sorely missed. She explained to me that she used to get frustrated and irritated by all the noise around her, but through meditation she has made peace with the noise because she says, "It is quieter inside now."

"Meditation can reintroduce you to the part of that's been missing."

—Russel Simmons

CHAPTER SIX

Movement and Yoga

"Do yoga in order to know what to do when you're not doing yoga."

—Rod Stryker

MOVEMENT... AS A yogi, you are familiar with movement, and likely have an affinity for it. Lucky you. Movement is essential for everyone, notwithstanding one's Doshic makeup. Movement increases circulation, drains lymphatic congestion, helps us expel toxins, nourishes the heart and lungs, perks up our metabolism, and stabilizes moods by releasing happy chemicals. Did you know the same chemical cocktail found in antidepressants automatically surges through our body when we exercise? The body is flooded with endorphins, oxytocin, serotonin, and dopamine as our heart beat and breath flows. The positive feeling of exercise is similar to morphine. If exercise is an unattractive word for you, don't think of it as exercise. Think of it as activity or a hobby. Exercising doesn't have to be a laborious event that involves a gym membership or bar bells. Basic movement such as walking, swimming, biking, and of course yoga are good for all three Doshas. Various activities will effect the Doshas in different ways. Just as food can be medicine for someone and poison for someone else, a certain activity can be conducive for someone, but potentially injurious for someone else. For example: cross-fit might be totally fine for a twenty-eight year old Kapha, but completely ill suited for a fifty-two year old Vata. Vata body types should minimize activities that amplify speed, or create a pounding effect of the joints. This is because Vatas are already quick and tend to have a more delicate frame. Vata types may gravitate towards running, but running can create an imbalance because quick plus quick, equals quicker. You recall, that we encourage more of the opposite to create balance. Vata types do well with grounding activities such as yoga, hiking, tai chi, and light weight lifting. Light weight lifting is especially important for people with a Vata constitution in the Vata stage of life, (50 years of age and older). We all lose bone density as we age, and the bone structure of Vata Dosha is already slight so they should strengthen their muscles. This is effective becomes bones grow stronger to support stronger muscles. Vata types should take care not to over do it. Something like cross-fit would not be advisable for a Vata body type because it is load baring and extreme for their slight frames.

Pitta types will feel most attracted to competitive sports, but highly competitive sports will irritate a Pitta person because the heat of the competition will exaggerate their natural tendency to push themselves towards perfectionism and triumph. Most likely, if you are a Pitta, you are goal oriented all day long. You thrive off productivity and perfectionism in your working life. Your form of exercise should balance out your magnetic tendencies towards hard work and acquiring accolades. Thrusting yourself into a competitive sport after a hards day work would be like drinking tabasco because you ate too many hot wings. We are looking for balance in order to feel our best. People with a Pitta constitution should do activities that are fun, lighthearted, cool, and calm. Yoga, kayaking, paddle boarding, skiing, surfing and swimming are some of the best activities for Pittas. Why? Because what puts out fire better than water? The tranquility of nature and waterscapes will escort Pittas into a contented and refreshed state of mind. Kapha types are strong and have endurance. Picture an NFL quarterback—Kapha. Some Kaphas may be resistant towards exercise because their slow, heavy, and dull qualities can gravitate more towards a couch, but it is essential to move. Kaphas are strong; they do well with more demanding activities such long distance or high intensity bike rides or runs. Kaphas can handle cross-fit, and do well with feisty activities like wrestling, kickboxing and martial arts. The emotional current of Kapha is sweet and calm, so the readiness and vigor required for contact sports illicit a balancing effect for Kapha Dosha. Spirited activities like bowling, horseback riding, golfing and such are safe for everyone. Just make sure the environment is not too hot or too cold, (extreme conditions provoke imbalances).

> *"The study of the asana is not about mastering posture. It's about using posture to understand and transform yourself."*
>
> **—B.K.S. Iyengar**

Yoga: My fellow yogi, you could have written this section. I am grateful to be in engaged with likeminded friends who are grateful for the castellations of positive benefits our yoga practices offer us each time we step onto our mats. Yoga provides us with a wide variety of movements and poses that can be performed to immaculately compliment each of our unique blueprints. Yoga has been around for thousand of years, common in the US since the 1950s, and has gained enormous leaps in recognition and popularity in the past decade. Yoga is one of the fastest growing industries in the United States. You and I both know yoga is absolutely more than an industry, and could never be diluted to the notorious image of a woman in downward facing dog, or lady in tree pose. We know yoga is not something we do, yoga is a lifestyle. When we refer to yoga in a Western context, we are usually speaking of asanas or postures. These physical poses help to strengthen, tone, lengthen, fortify, and preserve the body. Yoga may also bring you peace of mind, a sense of creativity, and connection. As you may recall, the word 'yoga,' means union. The essence is to unite with your True Nature. As you can see, the paramount theme of yoga at its core, is the same as Ayurveda—to return to your True Nature. Yoga and Ayurveda share themes and principles; Yoga is Ayurveda's sister science. Yoga is fantastic for everyone because there are a variety of styles and poses that can be selected, adapted, and modified to compliment everyone's mind-body constitution.

As a yoga teacher, people often ask, "How long did it take you to learn that?", or "How did you get so flexible?" I must admit, much of my flexibly and aptitude for asanas came naturally to me. I was a dancer when I was young and both my parents are oddly flexible. However, being bendy in no way, shape or form makes my practice better, stronger, or more advanced than anyone else's. I went to a class this morning and the teacher—Kelly said, "Now advance yogis only…Smile." Her humor was spot on. Being able to make a particular shape does not make one "advanced". Being able to listen to ones body, respect ones limitations and have a strong willingness to grow, while staying as peaceful as possible is far more impressive. Yoga, and this journey through life, is not about how impressive the container is. Whether it be the body, the house, the job, the car, the title ect.; this journey is about the contents within the container. We use Yoga and Ayurveda as tools to keep the body and mind healthy, and in doing so they are less likely to distract or detour us from our purpose. Ayurveda and Yoga help us to keep our vessels capable so that we can move through the world with more agility and mastery. If you are new to Yoga, please note that Yoga is not directly linked to any religious connotation. When I first started teaching, I taught in a gym where they told me, "Don't do that Omming thing because it scares people and this isn't a church or anything." I found that slightly humorous. I respected their wishes and vowed to help educate them as time progressed. Like Ayurveda, Yoga was born in Ancient India under the umbrella of Hinduism, but practicing Yoga does not require you to accept or subscribe to any particular belief system. By keeping your Doshas in balance, and by being a yogini, (a female yogi) you are not obligated to pray, step into a temple, learn about various Gods, chant songs, or do anything that you are no fully comfortable with. Ayurveda and Yoga are tools we put into our tool boxes. Our toolbox is like a treasure chest of ideas, applications, and essentials that help us feel good and function from a place of reverberating wellness.

> *"I do yoga two or three times a week. And by 'doing yoga' I really mean shaving my legs."*
>
> **—Anonymous**

Yoga Styles: As a yogi you may be well versed on the myriad styles of yoga available to us. I learned yoga in China, (and in Mandarin no less) so I had no clue as to what "style" I was enjoying, or that there were styles for that matter. I dove into Asthanga and trained in Hatha in India, but my mind was blown to learn of all the different styles that existed once I saturated myself into the yoga scene in the US. I'll tell you what, there is absolutely something for everyone. You may recall the moment you initially googled a yoga studio, checked out a yoga website, and walked into your first yoga class. You were introduced to foreign words like Namaste, Vinyasa, Hatha, Yin, and other terms that may have caused your brain to illuminate with question marks. As you invested more time into your practice these terms became familiar and relevant. I'm sure we share a fondness for the term Namaste. Namaste means, "The light within me honors, respects and supports the light in you". How sweet is that? Essentially, it expresses that I see you, I respect you, and I appreciate you. If it makes you feel more comfortable, think of it as Aloha. I gave two autistic girls private yoga lessons for years. I guided these sweet girls and their mother through yogic breathing, chants, and poses every-other week. One day, at the end of the practice I brought my hands to prayer and said, "Namaste." Alexa, the younger sister—immediately responded in complete reverence, "Aloha," as she too, placed her hands over her heart. She gets it. Incase you are newer to the yoga practice, study primarily at home, or in a studio that offers one specific style of yoga, you may be curious as to what else is out there. I'm providing a brief description of popular styles of yoga so that you can navigate your way into a studio or class that promotes the experience you may be seeking. The original form of physical yoga, (Asana) is called Hatha, meaning sun-moon. Hatha yoga balances our masculine and feminine qualities. This translates to making us both strong and active, yet also flexible and calm. Traditionally, Ayurveda speaks of Hatha yoga as a 'Chikitsa,' or treatment for many physical and mental imbalances. If you are new, or just want a 'feel good class', this is a great choice. Vinyasa Yoga means, "to place in a special way". The sequencing takes Hatha yoga postures and layers the breath and movement together to create a flow. This is a fun experience if you are in the mood to express yourself with your body. I find it to feel like a dance. Gentle/Basic Yoga: This style is geared towards beginners. The classes are thorough, slow and descriptive. Novice and veteran yogis benefit from gentle and basic classes. These classes provide a safe and supportive space for newbies to get their toes wet, and a great environment for experienced practitioners to revisit and fortify their foundation. Yin/Restorative Yoga: The postures are seated and held for longer durations of time, (1-5 minutes) Props such as blocks, blankets and straps are often utilized to provide support and comfort. The approach is therapeutic. As we touched on earlier, Yin and Yang are concepts from Chinese Medicine ; Ayurveda shares the same thought process. Yin is the perfect counterbalance to Yang. Yin is feminine, lunar and passive. Yang is masculine, solar and active. Regardless of our gender and Dosha, we all live Yang lives because Yang is the function of doing; as it seems modern times are times of doing. If you are on the go, you are in a Yang state. If you are stressed, you are in a Yang state. Almost all activities are Yang. Yang is the DO aspect of life, Yin is BE aspect of life. With that said, Yin is suitable and medicinal for everyone. I'd recommend you to try it if you haven't already. The benefits of Yin yoga enlist a similar effect as a glass of wine, (no joke). According to the Yin/Yang principle as applied to food and substances, wine is an expanding, or Yin substance. That is why drinking wine elicits relaxation. Power/Hot Yoga: This style produces heat and vigor. Power builds strength and stamina. Theses classes tend to be relatively intense. If you are an athlete, you probably gravitate towards this style because you are wired to be up for the challenge. The heat helps loosen stiff muscles. (Balance Power classes with Yin.) Ashtanga Yoga: The original Vinyasa. The primary sequence is designed to bring you endurance, strength, flexibility and balance. The sequencing is physically demanding; Ashtanga places a predominate emphasis on breath. Ashtanga is nice because it is the same sequence every time. Your muscles will start to memorize the sequences so you can keep your mind out of it and give attention to your breathing. This style can turn into a moving meditation. Bikram Yoga: 26 postures done in a heated room under strict direction. The sequencing opens the body and creates a balanced muscular-skeletal system. Bikram is unique in that you can do it in NYC, LA or Maui, and it will be the same exact 26 postures. All Bikam teachers are trained under uniform guidelines, so they all use similar language and cuing. Kundalini Yoga: From the Tantra school of Yoga—Kundalini uses poese, breath, meditation and chanting to awaken the "Kundalini" energy housed in the spine. The practice accesses the nerves system, glands and chakras. Some practitioners call this style, "the yoga of awareness."

"Go from a human being doing yoga, to a human being yoga."

—Baron Baptiste

Within these styles there is plenty of diversity. Yoga is not a one note song. Experiment. Try different studios and videos until you find what best suits you.You may notice that you gravitate towards a particular teacher more than a particular style. If your teacher is knowledgable, he or she can make almost any style pleasant for you by offering modifications and adjustments. The intention and energy of the teacher will color your experience; finding someone you resonate with will favor your experience. If your interest for yoga has been peaked, search for a local studio, then stop in and scope out the vibe. Online Yoga is available through sites like the Cody App and YogaGlo among others.

"Body is the bow, Asana is the arrow, Soul is the target."

—B.K.S. Iyengar

The Most Suitable Style per Dosha: The most suitable styles of yoga for Vata types are Hatha, Yin, Gentle, Restorative, and Bikram. These classes are offer a steady pace or slow rhthym. Bikram is good for Vata because Vata Dosha is cold, and Bikram is done in a heated room. This will create balance.Yoga styles that compliment Pitta Dosha are Hatha, Vinyasa Flow, (in AC—not hot), Yin, Restorative and Ashtanga. Yin and Restorative will help Pittas distress, while Hatha, Vinyasa and Ashtanga will all appease Pitta's natural athletic traits. Pittas should take caution in taking too many hot classes, (particularly in the summer). The best Yoga styles for Kapha Dosha are Power, Hot, Bikram, Ashtanga and Vinyasa. These styles will all incorporate sufficient movement and heat to break up the sedentary and cold qualities of Kapha Dosha. Kundalini Yoga would be good for anyone who feels compelled to practice it. Vata types will likely experience the waves of energy easily because they are sensitive. They should have a grounded and knowledgeable teacher there for support.

"Just shifting your ability to approach your yoga practice as a form of medicine can be really powerful."

—Tiffany Cruishank

Best Poses per Dosha: If you are newer to yoga, you will benefit from a teacher or video guide to help you identify these postures. A teacher will assist you through the poses and help you find the correct alignment, depth, and modifications as needed.

The seat or home of Vata is in the colon, that is why Vata types, or people with a Vata imbalance are prone to constipation. To balance Vata, the yoga practice should be grounding and have an emphasis on stimulating the colon and finding ease in the pelvis and low back area. Hip openers and prone, (face down) backbends are best. Frog, pigeon and child's pose are all excellent—along with sphinx, cobra and swan. Forward folds calm the nervous system, so standing or seated forward folds help to pacify Vata Dosha. Words carry a message, so for Vata types think of words like ground, slow, restore, relax, do less, stillness, stability, simple, heavy, dense, trust, earth, steady, warm, focus, sink, deepen, pause, supportive and rest.The seat or home of home of Pitta is in small intestine, that is why Pittas are susceptible to heartburn and acid indigestion. Backbends and twist help regulate Pitta and ring out excess bile. Side-bends help relieve excess heat from the internal organs. Bow, camel, wheel, seated and standing twists are all good. Pitta flows should have a cooling, fluid quality,(envision the feel of cascading waterfalls). Pittas should practice in an air conditioned environment. Optimal words for Pitta types are: cool, refresh, rejuvenate, relax, flow, renew, let go, patience, allow, softness, rivers, waterfalls, placid waters, tranquility, fluid, rinse, surrender, float, waves, play, receive and calm.

The home of Kapha is in the stomach and chest, (lung region). Poses that open the thoracic cavity, (rib cage area) help break up congestion and stagnation. Camel and half bridge are great. Twists are good because they detoxify sludge, or toxic buildup, and boost ones metabolism. Kapha sequencing should be dynamic, meaning the poses should not be stagnant. Holding poses for too long could put a Kapha is a sedentary zone. Movement is needed to counterbalance the slow and heavy qualities of Kapha. Kapha types will benefits from language like light, lighten up, energy, warmth, stimulate, detoxify, let go, forgive, melt, lift, bright, sweep, connect, motivate, move, travel, release, shed, free, illuminate, transfer, clear-out and clarity.

Most yoga poses are good for everyone as long as they are not done to the extreme. There should never be any pushing or force. For medicinal purposes, no one needs to wrap their foot behind their head or twist until they re-taste their lunch. If that sort of thing comes naturally and tickles your fancy—go for it. For the cornerstone aim of achieving balance, just explore the poses and styles that resonate with your True Nature.

How to choose the most suitable practice based on your Dosha and your day: Character Sketch: Meet Yogini Ashley: Ashley woke up at 7am and hit the ground running. She had a ton of calls, appointments, deadlines, and no lunch break. It's now 6pm and she's weaving through rush hour traffic in hopes to make it to her yoga studio by 6:30pm. There are two classes on the schedule for 6:30pm. She can take a Hot Power class, which will amp up her nervous system and require her muscles to click on and really work for her; or she can take a candlelight Restorative class, which will allow her to ground and relax. Which class should she choose? Keeping in mind that Ashley has had a long and stressful day, she should absolutely choose the Restorative option. This class will work as medicine for her mind and body.

Character Sketch: Meet Yogini Grace: Grace has had a wonderful weekend of pure relaxation. She spent the entire weekend in a hammock with the third book in her favorite trilogy. She enjoyed an ocean view, coconut ice cream and a cool breeze. As Sunday evening rolls around she decides it may be fun to take a yoga class. She looks on the schedule and sees there's a Hot Power class at her local studio. Is this a good option for Grace? Yes, why not? Grace has been lounging with ice cream in hand, a cool breeze against her skin, and a hammock under her tush all weekend. A little heat and vigor will stir-up anything that has become too cool or sedentary over the weekend. Great choice Grace!

PAUSE FOR AFFIRMATION

"I am committed to the practice that serves me."

A Balanced and Safe Sequence for Vata, Pitta and Kapha: Vatas should hold the poses for about five breaths. The stability of five breaths will ground Vatas tendency to move quickly. Pittas can hold the poses one or two breaths to eecouage a fluid quality. Kaphas can hold the poses for about three breaths. The slightly quicker sequencing will balance out Kaphas tendency to move very slowly.

Sun salutations (5-10 rounds)

Warrior 1

Warrior 2

Warrior 3

Step to the top of your mat. Mountain Pose

Chair Pose

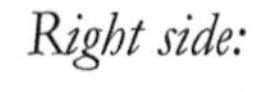

Right side:

Chair twist

Mountain

Tree Pose

Chair Pose

Left side:

Chair twist

Mountain

Tree Pose

Lie on belly

Sphinx

Cobra

Child's Pose

Lie on back

Half Bridge

(Can do wheel)

Reclined Spinal Twist

(Can do shoulder stand)

Corpse Pose

Short home practice to ground Vata Dosha

Child's pose—five breaths

Cobra pose—five breaths

Pigeon pose (right and left sides)—five breaths

Seated forward bend—ten breaths

Short home practice to refresh Pitta Dosha

Child's pose to Swan pose (back in forth in a fluid way five times)

Downward facing dog to up-dog (ripple forward and draw back like a wave)—five time

Step to top of mat—side bends (right and left)—3 times, 3 breaths each

Camel pose to open heart—five breaths

Reclined Twist (right and left sides)—3 breaths each side

Corpse pose—five minutes

Short home practice to stimulate Kapha Dosha

Cat-Cow pose—five times

Downward facing dog—three breaths

Step to top of mat—chair pose—three breaths

Chair twists (right and left sides)—three breaths

Lie down for bridge pose—five breaths

Supported reclined bound angel pose (boilster under mid-back to open chest)—10 breaths

Corpse pose—three minutes

CHAPTER SEVEN

Philosophy & Chakras

"Far better to live your own path imperfectly, than to live another's perfectly."

—Bhagavad Gita

THE FUNDAMENTAL PRINCIPLES of Yoga: I first traveled to India as a twenty-two year old girl with a pressing desire to learn how to contort into unique shapes. One day, my friends Kathy, Naomi and I, left the Ashram to walk down to the Ganga river. My friend Kathy's stomach began to hurt so bad that we almost had to turn around. She was grabbing her abdomen and kneeling over when a local man, with a long beard, turban, and a saffron colored scarf approached us. He said, "I am yogi. I help you." We were together, trusting, and felt safe. She lied down near the river and closed her eyes. The man placed his hands over her stomach, without touching her body. He closed his eyes and remained there for a short time. Naomi and I just looked at each other—curious, skeptical, and amused. A couple minutes later, the man removed his hand, Kathy opened her eyes and smiled. She got up and said she felt completely better. The man stepped down to the river, crouched towards the water and washed his hands .We thanked him. He wouldn't take money or payment for his help, but he kindly took a photo with us. And that was it. Kathy's pain was gone, so we continued our walk. During our time at the Ashram we walked down to the basement and listened to lectures offered by the leaders, or Gurus within the community. I bought several books on philosophy, spirituality, and the science of yoga. I watched closely as locals placed food in front of statues of Gods in temples, (known as Prasad), and listened to the waiter at the Ayurvedic restaurant near our Ashram describe how the food would bless us. I didn't understand any of it. But, I do remember the intrigue and interest that penetrated every cell in my body when I realized the scope of yoga was far broader than I presumed. The capacity to expand and to heal seemed to be available. I could almost taste the awe-inspiring experiences that would accompany that kind of journey if I was willing to take it. I was willing. I realized that an entire system of philosophy and theory lived within the science of yoga. I learned that the Asana practice is just one of eight electrifying limbs, or 'branches' of yoga .

"Yoga is 99% practice, and 1% theory."

—Sri Pattabhi Jois

Yoga is so much more than stretching, twisting, bending, and balancing on one precarious body part. Yoga postures are phenomenal in that they access every nook and cranny of our being. They open our Nadis, (channels of energy) and stimulate our Chakras,(reservoirs of energy). Chelsi, a good friend of mine and fellow yoga teacher, once said, "The act of teaching yoga is fascinating because we spend so much time cuing, referencing and talking about the physical, but the physical is just the route to access what yoga really is invisible. Yoga is sensation and energy." An asana, (posture) practice provides us with a vital-tangible route for learning about parts of ourselves that are, for all intents and purposes, invisible. Asana practices promote awareness, and awareness is the breeding ground for positive change. My friend Nicole says, "Every time I realize I have a problem, I immediately thank God for the awareness that I recognize the problem. Because without that awareness, I'd never have the sense to address it." Our practice is not exclusively for fixing, balancing, or improving ourselves, or any area of our lives. Our practice can highlight parts of ourselves we deserve to celebrate and enjoy! My friend Kelly says, "We are wonderfully imbalanced." It is true. Not every little thing needs to be fixed, manufactured, and fussed over. Sometimes it is more therapeutic to jubilantly embrace the wobbles, and appreciate the resilience that waits beneath the sway. Poses can be an outlet for creativity, expression, and playfulness. Practicing in a community and with friends can help strengthen relationships and promote connection. The most key aspect to our Asana practice is that it comes from the heart. Tony Robbins says, "Stay in your head, and you're dead." Our practice gives us an opportunity to shift from thinking to feeling; from analysis to intuition. As a yogi, you've experienced the ineffable laws of the practice that assure you—all is well in the world. The practice of showing up for yourself fully, free of judgment, and that neurotic self-critic is healing for the body, mind and heart. The amount of focus it takes to balance in the midst of wavering variables, like wobbly toes or unabated mental chatter requires that we become magnificently present. That kind of presence trains our minds to notice and nourish gratitude for the little things, (like our webbed fingers, and strong quads for instances), and more importantly that kind of presence spills over into every aspect of our daily lives. We become more balanced, less judgmental, more present, forgiving, and grateful on a moment to moment basis. These kinds of phenomenons happen as a byproduct of our Asana practice. Now that is a side effect I'm excited about. But Yoga is so much more than moving our bodies and creating shapes. It is an ancient philosophy, with a rich and comprehensive framework. Let's take a peek.

> *"Yoga should be practiced with insight and an uninterrupted heartbeat."*
>
> **—Bhagavad Gita VI.23**

The Branches or Limbs of Yoga Philosophy:

1. **Yamas:** Golden Rules. These or moral imperatives, they are essentially behaviors we should avoid.

2. **Niyamas:** Observances. These are basically virtuous habits and behaviors that we should include in our lives.

3. **Asanas:** Poses or postures, what we are familiar with in our yoga classes or home practice.

4. **Pranayama:** Expansion of life force through breath. We visited these techniques in the previous chapter. Pranayama is a wonderful tool for relaxation, disease prevention and cellular repair.

5. **Pratayahara:** As mentioned earlier, Pratayaha means expanding upon inner awareness as opposed to allowing external factors to consume our focus. This is practically applied by unplugging at night, so that we're not bombarded with high frequency blue light and stimulus that can disturb our sleep cycles. By meditating, you will naturally employ Pratayahara, or the withdrawal from the senses because we're not touching, tasting, smelling, (unless you're baking muffins) or looking around while meditating.

6. **Dharna:** Increase concentration. The root word of Dharna is Dhr which means, "to hold, maintain, keep." The ideas here is to hold or keep the mind on one particular state or focus on one particular subject. This happens intuitively when we are in a focused zone, whether it be at work, while creating an art project, engulfed in a meaningful conversation, or reading a book.

7. **Dhyana:** This literally means, contemplation or reflection. This is a state of meditation. Dharna leads to Dhyana. With Dharna, the mind is focused on one thing. While practicing Dhyana the mind is stable, and unwavering from thing to thing; there is no judgment, or presumptions about the one thing.

8. **Samadhi:** A state of ecstasy or transcending the self. This is sometimes called Nirvana (not the band from the 90's). This is a state of enlightenment, or the highest degree of self -awareness. Samadi is described as the place where there is no separation between the the one who meditates, the act of meditating and the subject of meditation. Everything absorbs into everything else and there is no separation. Jesus, Buddha, Allah, Krishna, among others have reached Samadhi.

"Truth is the same always. Whoever ponders it will get the same answer. Buddha got it. Patanjali got it. Jesus got it. Mohammed got it. The answer is the same, but the method of working it out may vary this way or that."

—Swami Satchiotananda

Yamas and Niyamas are the first two limbs of yoga philosophy. We will dive a bit deeper into these principles because they offer a moral skeleton for an enriched life. I think of the Yamas and Niyamas as simply as the proverbial, "Everything you needed to learn, you learned in kindergarten." Whether you are five, thirty-five or eighty-five years old, obtaining success, status, and praise feels good—but the air comes right of the balloon if you had to cheat or connive to get your way there. Ultimately, the things that are most fulfilling are born of authenticity. The Yamas and Niyamas remind us of concepts that we may have forgotten or glossed over through the course of our lives; they revive our eagerness to practice everything we learned in kindergarten. I've included exercises to help you assimilate the ideas into your daily life as you see fit.

The Yamas and Niyamas. Yamas, are the first limb of yoga philosophy, and they represent restrictions, or acts we should avoid because they go against virtues. There are five Yamas:

» Ahisma, means non-harming in action, thought, word or deed. Non-harming applies to yourself, others and our planet. Integrate Ahisma into your life by treating yourself well. Allow a kind voice to drive your inner monologue.

Practice: *You can practice Ahisma by replacing any negative thought towards yourself with the exact opposite thought. For example, if someone is explaining something to me and I don't understand, my inner critic mights think, "You're dumb. You'll never get it." That thought is harmful, (and inaccurate). I will practice Ahisma towards myself by immediately replacing that old false script with a new story. "I am intelligent. I am capable of understanding."*

» Aparigraha, means non-hoarding. This relates to attachment to relationships, experiences and possessions. Non-hoarding also relates to not withholding your gifts, greatness or ultimate potential. Your talents were given to you with the intention of you using them towards a collective contribution. Your talents were bestowed upon you with the intention of you utilizing them for the greater good. Share your gifts!

Practice: *Create a list of talents, skills or qualities that you possess that will be of value when you apply them to help other people. Brainstorm ways that you can harness your skillets to directly impact the life of someone else. For example, if you're a talented writer, can you proofread a book for a friend? If you're fantastic at organizing, can you assist your neighbor with rearranging her garage? If you are a patient person, can you step aside and let the person behind you in line go first since they seem to be in a hurry? Sometimes it is tricky to recognize your own gifts because they come so naturally to you, you may not even see them as special. Feel free to ask friends and family members to help identify your gifts. Never trivialize your gifts. You are here to make a unique stamp on the world...Aparigraha would suggest you not withhold that.*

» Asteya, means non-stealing. This does not only apply to obvious things like stealing goods or manipulating the use of services. Asteya can also be in the form of setting exceedingly high expectations, and robbing yourself or others of the chance to feel satisfied or accomplished. Non-stealing includes wasting someone's time and energy, or allowing someone to be a thief of your precious time and energy.

Practice: *Take a gentle scan of your heart. Is there someone in your life who is depleting your energy by taking up space with unrealistic expectations, or taking advantage of your time? (I have referred these people referred to as 'energy vampires'.) Can you distance yourself from this person? Wayne Dyer says, "If you meet someone who's soul is not aligned with yours, send them love and move along."*

» Brahmacarya, is not being wasteful with our energy. This applies to not over extending ourselves, not thrusting our agendas onto others, and not absorbing the energy of others if it is not conducive to our True Nature and path.

Practice: *Look at your calendar, can you identify spaces in your schedule where you are stretching yourself too thin? Ask yourself these questions: Is this necessary? Is this helpful? Can this be done another time? Can I create space for rest?*

» The final Yama is Satya, or honesty. Being truthful to ourselves and others allows us to align with our higher purpose with less interference and more clarity. Practice: For twenty-four hours monitor your correspondences, conversations and inner monologue. Can you spot any white lies, exaggerations or omissions? Don Miguel Ruiz is the author of *The Four Agreements.* In his book he shares with us his four core virtues: Never take anything personally, always do your best, don't make assumptions, and be impeccable with your word. See if for twenty-four hours, you can be impeccable with your word. This is a practice of Satya.

"Never producing pain by though, word and deed, in any living being, is what is called Ahimsa, non-injury"

—Swami Vivekananda

The second limb of yoga, the Niyamas highlight areas of our lives and character that should be accentuated.

» The first is Santosha, or contentment. Santosha encourages you to be happy where you are, enjoy who you are with, and be okay with your current circumstances no matter what they may be. We have a tendency to constantly want to improve, do more, and do better. A healthy sense of advancement is good so long as we see the value in where we already are. Kapahs have a natural affinity to Santosha because they are easy going, whereas Pittas struggle with Snatosha because they are so driven. Practice: Meditation is the easiest way to practice Santosha. Sit and be.

» Svadhya, or self-study is a big one for me, probably my favorite in the bunch. Self-study includes learning to understand ourselves, taking time for reflection, reading texts that provide wisdom and insight, and learning how to apply the takeaways into our own lives.

Practice: *Ayurveda is founded on the premise that self-study equates to self-healing. Reading this book and engaging yourself in the process is a courageous act of Svadhya. Kudos to you my friend.*

» Sauca, means cleanliness. This is to have a clean and pure body, (fresh food, exercise and hygiene), a pure mind, (minimal negative or hostile thoughts), and a pure heart (less resentment—more love). Sauca encourages us to be mindful and deliberate with what we allow into our environment, mind, and body.

Practice: *Next time you sit down for a meal, observe your mindset. What are you thinking about? What are you eating? How is the environment you are eating in? What does it look and smell like? What kind of conversation are you having while you eat? Are you watching TV or working? What are you watching? What are you working on? You don't need to "change" anything. Raising your awareness as to what is currently happening with help you assess if something in your life would benefit from becoming more pure. According to Ayurveda, when we eat, we are not only ingesting and assimilating the food, we are also digesting the thoughts and impressions of entire experience. We all eat, so we all have a chance to practice Sauca three times a day. Mealtimes offer a great point in the day to narrow in on the content of what we are digesting—food, thoughts, and the environment in that given moment.*

» Tapas, means discipline, zest, or austerity. This applies to putting in the work ; Tapas is to be committed to the task, the journey, and the work it takes to see it through. Tapas implies that we should preserver through struggles, awkwardness, pains, and vulnerable points. Essentially, Tapas reminds us to stay the course. Pittas are great with Tapas because they are ambitious. Vatas struggle with Tapas because they loose focus and lack a natural tendency to follow through. Kaphas in a state of balance can endure, so long as they stay motivated. Rumi says, "Success is the ability to get from one failure to another without loosing enthusiasm." The etymology of 'enthusiasm' comes from the Greek idea of, "the God within." I think when we set out to accomplish, achieve, try, or experience something new, great, or exciting it comes from a place of enthusiasm. The impetus—in every sense of the word, comes from the God within. It is our duty to preserve the God within—that space in us that knows I am able, I can and I will. The practice of Tapas is the practice of persevering and honoring the God within.

Practice: *Solute the ways you are currently practicing Tapas. Have you been meditating daily? Did you make a commitment to thin out your schedule and give yourself more time to rest and restore? Have you been choosing yoga classes that balance your Dosha? Have you made significant changes in your life despite set backs and hurdles? Have you been consistent with this? If so, you are using discipline, you are feeding your zeal. Congratulations to you!*

» The final Niyama is, Isvara Pranidhana. This means surrender to God. Do what you can with what you have, give it your all with sincerity and gall, then release the results. Give your worries, your pains, your apprehensions, your faults, your errors, your good tidings, your strengths, and your gifts to God, (or the universe, light, the greater good…whatever you choose to name it). Offer up all you have, all that's holding you back, and all that's moving you forward—then trust the intelligent design of the universe, or bigger picture to do its part -knowing you did yours. Practice: For me the easiest way to practice Isvara

> Pranidhana is to trust. This week if you feel anxious, stress, or confused i'd welcome you to pray and trust. You can even say, "I am Trust. I am Trust. I am Trust." Write in on sticky notes for your a mirror, computer, and datebook. The Serenity Prayer embodies and beautifully expresses this concept. "God, grant me the serenity to accept the things I cannot change, courage to change the things I can, and wisdom to know the difference."

If your interest has been peaked you can access a wealth of information and depth on the eight limbs of Yoga in the Y*oga Sutras,* written by Patanjali. This book was compiled in 400CE. The book gained popularity when a revered Indian Guru by the name of Swami Vivekananda came to the US as a teacher in the late 1900s. The Yoga Sutras can be found easily online or in a bookstore.

"Everything in life pulsates with energy, and all of this energy contains information."

—Caroline Myss

"Chakras are organizational centers for the reception, assimilation, and transmission of life-force energy. They are stepping stones between heaven and earth."

—Andrea Judith

Chakras, and understanding the invisible laws of energy: Chakras are not some new age, hipster term to be tossed around to explain why you're always late, or why your best friend is grouchy.

I've had adorable friends say to me, "Sorry I'm late my first Chakra is out of balance," and, "Gosh, I must be cranky because my heart Chakra feels neglected." While these comments are cute, and potentially accurate, there is much more to Chakras than black and white correlations. I do not profess to be an expert on Chakras. I do however, find them fascinating, and felt compelled to share what I know with you. The clinical professor at George Washington University Medical Center stated in the 2005 journal of *Evidence-Based Complimentary Alternative Medicine* that,"Subtle energy forms both inform and transcend the faculties of the five senses. They are taken into the body via openings called Chakras, and translate into a form of energy the body can use, literally use, at a cellular level just as the pineal is the energy transducer for environmental information, the Chakras are energy transducers for subtle energy. Subtle energy is healing energy that anyone can learn to perceive and utilize. It is crucial, but often a missing component in health care." You have likely realized that when exploring this system of mind-body medicine it is important to keep in mind that Eastern traditions do not rely solely upon things that can be seen and touched to explain health and disease. So much of Ayurveda and yoga deal with energetics, which happen to be in the realm of the unseen. Our Western minds are accustomed to accepting things we can see, touch, and measure, but there is far more than meets the eye. There is an entirely more subtle component to our wellbeing. It is an energetic system. You know this because we cannot completely see or touch Vata, Pitta, and Kapha. At this time, I cannot hook you up to a machine to measure how much Pitta is saturating your liver or how much Kapha is in your lungs. I cannot look into your imaginative mind and tell you just how much Vata is there, but you know Vata, Pitta, and Kapha are always present despite our inability to physically see or touch them. In congruence with the Doshas and qualities, there are the Nadis, (channels of energy) and Chakras, or wheels of energy. The Chakras represent bundles of nerve endings, organs and emotions. The Chakras run up the spine or Central Channel of the body. There are seven main Chakras that run from the tailbone up to the crown of the head. Each Chakras is bubbling with specific functions and vitality. Prana flows through the channels and through the Chakras. It is useful for us to keep the Chakras open, because if a Chakra is closed than the energy is blocked. Blocked energy leads to imbalanced Doshas. Think of your Central Channel or spine as a large hose—if a Chakra is closed then there is a kink in the hose and there is a halt in the flow of energy. We want flow. Flow equates to maximum Prana flooding our channels and coursing through our veins. This is a good thing! We discussed how breath, meditation, yoga, whole foods, and nature help us access and harness maximum Prana. We know stress depletes us of Prana. Keeping our Chakras open is another way to protect our Prana and our health. Keeping your Doshas balanced will naturally help open and safeguard your Chakras. Opening your Chakras is not as easy as opening your favorite story book or jar of jam. Chakras are convergence points for the mind, body, and soul. When something effects the emotional sphere, it effects the physical sphere as well. For example, Lauren was going through a divorce when she became extremely sad and heartbroken. During this time she developed a respiratory infection. Her heartburn returned for the first time in years, and her chest was tender to the touch. The emotional impact of the divorce manifested in the Heart Chakra area of her body.

Let's have a look at the Seven Chakras:

The first Chakra, or root Chakra is called, Muladhara. This area of the body represents stability, security, and our basic survival needs. It encompasses the first three vertebra, the bladder, and colon. When this Chakra is functioning well—we feel fearless. The first Chakra, or root is associated with the element, Earth. The Earth element shares a connection to Kapha Dosha. You'll recall, the word Kaphas means, "That which holds things," and the root is what holds the tree in place. Kapha and the root Chakra both symbolize stability. Signs that your first Chakra may be out of balance include: feeling unsafe, feeling financially insecure, feel, "stuck," or unable to move forward in life, and feeling disconnected from people and the environment around you. Physical issues from the root of your spine down to the soles of your feet, as well as adrenal, bone and immune issues are indicative of a root Chakra imbalance. A positive affirmation to nurture your root Chakra is, "I am safe and secure. I am provided for." You will know your root is solid when you feel safe, abundant, connected and seated in yourself and the way you're living your life. To help balance your root Chakra include poses such as child's pose, hero's pose and easy seat, or lotus in your yoga practice.

The second Chakra, or sacral Chakra is called Svadhisthana. This area governs our creativity and sex drive. Svadhisthana is located in the space of our reproductive organs. When this Chakra is open we feel creative and passionate about creating the life we want and creating new life (this correlates with the libido). The elemental make up of the second Chakra is Water, here elementally there is a connection to both Pitta (fire and water) and Kapha (earth and water).Vatas are the creative ones and Svadhisthana governs creativity, so the second Charkra has an affinity to Vata Dosha as well. Your sacral Chakra may be out of alignment is you: have a hard time expressing yourself, engage in meaningless sexual encounters, feel like you're not "creating the life you want," feel like you have to fulfill the role of being sexy, hot or flirty to be accepted, experience reoccurring creativity blocks or "writers block" for example. Physically, a second Chakra imbalanced could manifest as issues with the reproductive organs, yeast infections, STDs, or reoccurring urinary tract infections. A positive affirmation to balance your second Chakra is, "I am creating the life I want and deserve." You'll know your second Chakra is aligned when you feel creative, able to engage in meaningful sexual and emotional relationships, confident in your ability to design the life you want, sound in your ability to express yourself freely, and can easily reveal your highest self to others. To help promote proper flow in the area of your second Chakra integrate dancing lion, pelvic titles and standing pelvic circles, and frog pose into your yoga practice.

The third Chakra, or solar plexus Chakra is called Manipura. This Chakra is located in the solar plexus area, right above the navel. This is the area of ambition, drive, and self-esteem. When this Chakra is open we feel confident and ready to tackle our dreams. Manipura is associated with Fire, as is Pitta. The third Chakra lends itself to an ambitious state, as does Pitta Dosha. Your third Chakra may need attention if you are easily irritated, obsessed with accomplishments, controlling, questioning your self-worth, or feeling powerless. Physically, an imbalance in the third Chakra could express itself as digestive issues, gallbladder issues, ulcers, constipation or heartburn. A positive affirmation is boost your third Chakra is, "I am radiant and call forth my highest self." You will know you have achieved balance in this area when you feel motivated, cooperative, nonjudgemental, and inspired to reach your goals for the benefit of the greater good. To fuel your third Chakra incorporate seated spinal twists, bow pose and side bends into your practice.

The fourth Chakra is Anahata, and it is located in the heart. This Chakra is the meeting point for our lower three Chakras, (considered more physical) and our higher Chakras,(considered more spiritual). This area governs love, compassion, and forgiveness. The heart Chakra is the bridge for the body, mind, and spirit. The heart Chakra is linked to the element, Air. Characteristically, there is a connection between Vata and the heart Chakra. This shows up in practical terms because Vatas tend to be more sensitive to other people's emotions and empathic. Your fourth Chakra may need care if you: resist other people's love, have a hard time expressing love, dislike physical contact, feel resentful, are holding a grudge, feel a loss of joy. Physical manifestations include, tightness in the chest, breast or heart pains, issues with breathing, or extreme adversity to touch. A positive affirmation to heal the heart Chakra is, "I am loved. I am loving. Love is all there is." You will know your heart Chakra is balanced when you feel compassion for others, a generous dose of self-love, able to let grievances go, enjoy the company and contact of others, and value emotional intelligence and the ability to understand and respect peoples feelings. To help nourish your heart Chakra include camel pose, wheel pose and bridge pose in your daily asana practice.

The fifth Chakra, or throat Chakra is called Vishuddha. It is located near the throat and governs expression, self-knowledge, and our ability to speak our truth. The thyroid, parathyroid, jaw, neck, and tongue are all related to Vishuddha. Your fifth Chakra may be imbalanced if you are: lying, feeling "chocked up," unable to listen, constantly interrupting others, using spiteful words or not feeling confident in your message. An imbalance in the fifth Chakra could show up as reoccurring sore throats, change in vocal tone, TMJ, laryngitis, thyroid or parathyroid issues. A positive affirmation to heal the throat Chakra is, "I am expressing myself. I am understood. I am hearing the expression of others. I am understanding." You'll know you're more balanced when you can effectively communicate, speak truthfully and with conviction, seek truth and understanding, and are forthright with your honest thoughts and feelings. To help open your throat Chakra bring fish pose, shoulder stand and camel pose (with your head draped back) into your yoga practice.

The sixth Chakra, or third-eye Chakra is called Ajna. Ajna is located at the space between our eye brows. This is the seat of our intuition. When this Chakra is open we are able to gather insights and trust our instincts. Ajna is associated with ether or space, and has an affinity to Vata Dosha. Vata and Ajna share a receptivity to insight and intuition. Your sixth Chakra may need attention if you: are not feeling like you can trust your gut, are not following your instincts, have difficulty making life decisions, suffer from depression or mood swings, or unable to concentrate. A positive affirmation for strengthening the third-eye Chakra is, "I am connected to the infinite source of wisdom and knowledge we all share." You will know you're third eye is balanced when you trust your gut, access knowledge from meditation and divine practices, can focus on the task at hand for the benefit of the whole, feel inspired to live your life with purpose and make decision without much hesitation. To inspire a brighter sixth Chakra try headstand and shoulder stand with an inner gaze toward the third eye.

The seventh Chakra, or crown Chakra is Sahaswara and it is located on the crown of the head. This is the area of enlightenment of spiritual connection. When this Chakra is open we feel connected to the sun, moon, stars, humanity and the divine. When this Chakra is open we feel our life has purpose and meaning.

The seventh Chakra is also linked to the etheric or Vata realm. Your seventh Chakra may need care if you: always feel a need to defend you beliefs, are overly cynical and skeptical, are devoid of inspiration, resist learning new information or seeing things from a different perspective, are bored with life and feel malaise no matter what you do. Seventh Chakra imbalances range from nervous system and degenerative disorders to hormone imbalances and severe depression. "I am here for a reason. I am revealing my unique purpose." You will know you crown Chakra is balanced when you feel confident in your beliefs, willing to accept other people's beliefs, inspired to live a meaningful life, willing to explore new vantage points, present on a moment to moment basis, connected to God or something higher than yourself, an ambassador of peace and eager to help others. To access your seventh Chakra practice easy seat or lotus pose while focusing on your third eye in meditation. Rabin pose and headstand are also beneficial.

There is not an A+B=C equation as to how the Chakras and Doshas configure. Sometimes there will be an obvious or direct correlation, and sometimes there will not. I look at these concepts the way I look at ingredients. Somethings just go well together, like salt and pepper. That doesn't mean I have to use salt when I use pepper or that pepper is useless without salt. It doesn't mean I must utilize every ingredient I have to make a dish. These concepts come with a freedom to explore and dabble. Similar to the Doshas, cultivating an awareness around the Chakras will give you a broader vantage point and additional clues when something needs to be addressed. At this point, you can consider yourself a wellness detective. Open yourself to the vast world of introspection. Inquire within. Give yourself the time and space, free of distractions, so that you can hear your internal wisdom and proceed as your inner wisdom requests.

"What drains your spirit drains your body. What fuels your spirit fuels your body."

—Caroline Myss

We can balance our Chakras with Sound and Meditation: Each Chakras has a corresponding sound and color. Chakras are bundles of energy and fields of vibration. Color and sound both carry vibrations that help align the vibrations in our Chakras. For this meditation you can sit up tall or lie down flat, (if sitting is not an option). Just make sure your spine is as straight as possible and make sure that you feel comfortable. If you're sitting, sit up tall. Feel rooted in the hips, and lift long through the spine. Feel the long line from the tail bone up through the crown of the head. Allow your shoulders to fall away from the ears, and feel your chin is running level with the earth. Assure that you are not slouching or jetting your chin up to the sky. Envision the spine and each Chakra illuminated along the spinal column. Beginning at the base and working your way up to the crown see the root Chakra as the color RED, the sound here is LAM. See the color RED and chant the sound LAM seven times.

Draw your awareness up the spine to the second Chakra. The color is Orange and the sound is VAM. Visualize the color orange at the space of the reproductive organs and chant the sound VAM seven times.

Journey your awareness up to the third Chakra. The color is YELLOW and the sound is RAM. See the color yellow at the solar plexus and chant the sound RAM seven times.

Continue up the spine to the forth Chakra. The color is GREEN and the sound is YAM. See the color GREEN flood the heart and chant the sound YAM seven times.

Follow the spine up to the fifth Chakra as the throat. The color is BLUE and the sound is HUM. Envision the color blue at the throat and chant HUM seven times.

Rise up the spine to the sixth Chakra at the space between the eyebrows. The color is INDEGO and the sound is OM. See the color INDEGO and chant the sound OM seven times.

Grow all the way up to the seventh Chakra on the crown of the head. The color is VIOLET and the sound is a silent OM, (like an echo). Draw your awareness to the crown of your head, see the color VIOLET and chant OM silently, (in your mind) seven times.

Character Sketch: Meet Monica: Monica is an attorney. She dreads going to work. She knows her work environment drains her because there is a high level of drama in her work environment. Her associates are currently being vindictive. The atmosphere is cut throat. She would rathe not work there, but as of yet, Monica hasn't secured a replacement position at a different firm. She tries to keep the peace by biting her tongue at work every day. She just wants to make it through until a new job appears. A few weeks ago Monica developed a sore throat. She drank hot water with lemon and nursed it, but it didn't get better. This week it turned into laryngitis. She can barely talk. Monica didn't feel free to express herself and speak her truth at work. The implications of the, "Cut throat environment" caused her to, "Bite her tongue". These emotional blocks manifested physically in her fifth Chakra. The throat Chakra—the same one that governs free expression. It would be useful for Monica to balance and protect her throat Chakra. She can alleviate and prevent future physical pain by gargling salt water with turmeric and then licking honey. Monica wishes take care of herself by finding a new job, practicing home remedies like the ones mentioned above, and by learning how to balance and protect her energetic systems. Since Monica displays an imbalance in the fifth Chakra, she can focus on the fifth Chakra by envisioning the color blue and chanting the sound HUM seven times morning, noon, and night or by chanting HUM 108 times as she goes around a strand of Mala beads. Mala beads are a strand of 108 beads that are used for a type of meditation called, Japa meditation. Monica could hold the beads in between her pointer finger and thumb and chant HUM on each bead. By the time she goes around the entire strand, she will have chanted HUM 108 times. This type of meditation charges the beads with her intention so that overtime, as she touches the beads she will receive a stronger thread of support. The Japa meditation will sharpen her energetic ability to replenish her throat Chakra. Monica could also layer a Mantra, (mind-training) into her Chakra balancing practice. She could repeat to herself, "I am heard. I am understood. I am truth" when she wakes up and goes to sleep at night. As we have experienced, stating something in the, "I AM" form gives it quality of absoluteness. By reiterating this to herself and the universe on a daily basis, she is making it clear to the universe that she is receptive to a shift in the situation or in her perspective.

Character Sketch: Meet Michelle: Michelle and her husband were living paycheck to paycheck. Her husband John had recently lost his job, so they are down to a single source of income. Michelle was feeling a lot of pressure regarding their financial insecurity. She was clipping coupons and buying staple items like rice and beans in bulk to cut costs. Michelle became constipated. She only had a bowel movement once a week, and even then it is dry, hard, and required a painful push to get any release at all. Michelle's root Chakra was out of balance. The emotional stress around not feeling financially stable manifested in the colon, (root Chakra area of the body). I suggested to Michelle that when she wakes up each morning she should go sit next to her bamboo tree on her patio, and chant the sound for her first Chakra. Michelle took to this idea with optimism.(She is Vata Dosha, so she's easily excitable…and prone to constipation). She decided to replant her bamboo in a red, (color of the first Chakra) pot and chant LAM seven times every morning. By the third day Michelle texted me to tell me she had a regular bowel movement. She texted me every day that week to share that she was continuing the meditation and her bowels were regular. She was very relieved.

Do not be alarmed if you can't see the color. Sometimes you have to stretch your imagination a little and relax into it for it to appear. There is a stunningly massive amount of history and theory behind each of these concepts. This is not a curriculum style text book. There is no exam. You do not need to commit to this school of thought. My guess is, if you've made it this far in the book you are a seeker who is receptive to thoughts that stretch the boundaries of mainstream thinking. Continue to be curious. Continue to be fascinated. Magic resides in these faculties. Albert Einstein said, "I have no great talent, I am only passionately curious." If you're interested in Chakras and how they translate into mind-body medicine I would recommend "The Spirit of Anatomy" by Caroline Myss.

Eastern and Western Medicine Alignment... Several years ago, my mom was suffering from TMJ issues, a imbalance in the jaw that creates tension and pain. During this same time period, she noticed a drastic change in her voice. Her voice dropped several octaves over the course of the year. When she went to the doctor to address these concerns, they identified the issues as separate entities, concluding that TMJ is caused by stress and the voice change can be attributed to fluctuations in hormones. According to Ayurveda and the science of Yoga, the two separate issues were not separate at all. They are both signals that the throat Chakra was out of balance. Interestingly enough, my mom came home to tell me that the TMJ specialist requested she "sing" the sound "HUM" everyday. My eyes lit up as I immediately connected that Western Medicine verified the validity of sound and vibration healing. The same sound "HUM" was recognized as the healing sound for the same area of the body over 3,000 years prior. Regardless of the modality, in the end—medicine is intended to heal the patient. And sometimes Eastern and Western, new and ancient, meet on the very same page, with the very same conclusion.

PAUSE FOR AFFIRMATION

"I am aligned with the flow of the universe that flows through me."

Practice: *If you are currently experiencing an imbalance—identify what Chakra the imbalance is associated with. Incorporate the healing affirmation, yoga pose (s), and/or sound and color meditation into your daily routine. Observe how by directing your attention and intention to this area of the body the disharmony becomes more harmonious. If you see an improvement, continue the healing practice until the issue is resolved and you regain complete balance in that area of the body.*

EAT FOR YOUR CHAKRAS

Root Chakra: EARTH—RED

Root vegetables, carrots, potatoes, sweet potatoes, yams, squash, ginger, radishes and parsnips. Dense foods that contain high concentrations of the earth element: nuts, seeds and legumes. Red foods: cherries, tomatoes, radishes, beets, strawberries and red bell peppers.

Sacral Chakra: WATER—ORANGE

Due to the water element of the second chakra, fluids are key: hot teas, warm water and golden milk. Juicy fruits such as oranges, pineapples and mangoes are great. All other orange foods: turmeric, orange bell peppers, carrots, tangerines and peaches are perfect.

Solar Plexus Chakra: FIRE—YELLOW

Located in the home of your Agni, heating foods that stimulate your Agni are best. Try cayenne, ginger, black pepper and Agni Spices. Fiber rich foods will prevent stagnation in the third chakra—roughage like kale and broccoli, apples, beans and flaxseed are great for keeping things moving. The color of this chakra is yellow, so yellow foods such as lemon, yellow red peppers, bananas and grains like quinoa are great.

Heart Chakra: AIR—GREEN

Green foods carry the energy of the heart—try leafy greens, brussel sprouts, green cabbage, green apples, book choy, snow peas, green lentils and sea algae like chlorella.

Throat Chakra: ETHER—BLUE

Soups with sea vegetables, like Miso soup with seaweed nurtures the throat.

Third Eye Chakra: no direct element—Indigo

Reduce caffeine and stimulates, they cloud the third eye. Drugs and sedatives impair the third eye. Golden milk protects the third eye. Purple foods such as berries, purple kale, purple potatoes, plums and figs are great.

Crown Chakra: no direct element—Violet

A variety of simple, pure, Prana rich foods

> *"Keep Calm and Eat the Rainbow!"*
>
> **—Anonymous**

Poem…

When the world around us crumbles to its knees, we will stand on our feet.

And we will proclaim together that we have chosen to be here,

Committed here to what shakes us, sculpts us, and emboldens us to be,

Be fully human.

Perfectly flawed.

Flawed in ways that keep us humble and growing.

Growing to be inspired, empowered, empathetic, and kinder.

Kindness being our greatest strength.

And for those of us who have fallen, who choose to remain on our knees,

We are not weak.

We have chosen for the moment to be closer to the earth.

A pause to connect to her richness, the fullness, to be filled up, to be lifted,

To rise again.

Again, when the world quivers,

We will all stand.

Stand for what makes us smile, what makes the heart sing, what gives us wings.

Wings to fly above fear.

Fear that is small compared to our love.

Love that is timeless and endless.

Demands nothing.

Gives to all.

And laughs.

Laughs because it's infectious in its healing.

And joyful with the relief it imparts.

Imparting reminders of wholeness to anyone who feels incomplete.

Complete now.

In thanks, to a good earth and gods peace.

CHAPTER EIGHT

Self-Care & Daily Routines

"Drop the idea of becoming someone. For you are already a masterpiece. You cannot be improved. You have only to come to know it, to realize it."

—Osho

"How can you quench someone else's thirst if your cup is empty?"

— Christiane Northrup

PROVIDING OURSELVES WITH sufficient self-care is the most potent way to use life as medicine. Self-care is synonymous with self-love. It is the heartbeat, the very breath of how we are able to make a sustainable stamp on this world. I find self-care is the most overlooked, yet essential form of medicine. Self-care wraps it's loving arms around everything we have talked about so far… self-knowledge, stress management, nature, whole foods, breathe, movement and meditation. Integrating these nourishing items and activities into our lives is a way of practicing self-care.

Self-care request that you make yourself a priority rather than an afterthought. Self-care asks that when you make a list of everyone you love in this world, your name comes high on that list. Self-care is self-love and recognizes that every other love is an extension of the love we have for ourselves. Much of our striving, catering, working, and giving is an appendage of our inner most desire to love and be loved in return. We must love ourselves first. Giving is good, but we can only give what we have. We must nourish ourselves with an attentiveness and care that matches what we want to extend to others. I've been to many Statsangs, or spiritual gathering or discourses in both India and the US. It's funny because when the Guru or leader opens the forum for questions and answers, it seems to be no matter what the question is the Guru will respond, "Just meditate." I find it equal parts humorous and true. An exceptional publishing house that publishes renowned books on motivation, spirituality, and health, HayHouse Publishing is operated by a ninety-year old woman named Louise Hay. She is a spectacular woman with the spirit of a child and health and charm of a lady in her prime. She reminds me of the Gurus because she has a singular cure for every ailment too. Hers is, "Love Yourself". You are tired. Love Yourself. There's a controversy at work. Love Yourself. Your kids are acting out. Love Yourself. You were diagnosed with a disease. Love Yourself. You are always late. Love Yourself. No matter what the disturbance, her advice is as simple as it is profound—Love Yourself. Nowadays, many of us wear multiple hats and juggle several roles. It's vital for the sake of your health and sanity to carve out time for you. Everything is interconnected with everything else. If we deplete the earth's resources, we will be depleted. If we neglect ourselves, we neglect the whole. The enormity to which this entanglement extends is both alarming and enlightening. Making yourself a priority does not take away from anyone else. Everything you do for yourself is a reflection and catalyst for everything you are able to do for others. Self-care is not a luxury. Self-care is a necessity.

"Self-care is not about indulgence. It's about self-preservation."

—Audrey Lorde

Carve out time for yourself. What makes your heart sing? You can be creative in this department. It is not uncommon to erroneously drape guilt over the act of taking time for ourselves. This guilt is senseless and wasteful. Guilt leaks Prana. Retain your Prana. Your family, coworkers and friends will be delighted to see your batteries recharged after periods of care. Returning happier and rejuvenated will increase your productivity. Our energy is contagious. If bad habits and disease can be infectious, good habits and health are just as, if not more so, contagious. Taking care of yourself just may inspire those around you to take care of themselves too.

What's the difference between self-care and selfishness, or primping? A student politely raised her hand and asked this question during one of my Ayurveda trainings. I appreciate this question because I think it's important to clarify the distinction between self-care for the benefit of soul and wellbeing, and self-care for the benefit of ego, or vanity. The self-care we encourage in Ayurveda is focused on protecting, restoring, and revitalizing our energy. When our energy is balance by means of such self-care we can effectively contribute to a collective sense of wellbeing towards ourselves and everyone we encounter. While the physical body is a vessel for our soul, and the main outlet in which our energy animates—the physical body is a means, not the end. If our intentions behind our self-care practices are only about caring for the physical body, we have likely become distracted by the means and forgot the end. Focusing on the physical body isn't a bad thing. It's our most tangible outlet and barometer to our energy body. We just want to make sure that whatever it is we choose to incorporate into our self-care practices benefits and balances our energy, not just makes us feel, "pretty". For example, if I chose to get a pedicure, I want to appreciate the time as a point in my life where I can give myself permission to relax, breathe, and receive. Getting a pedicure because I want my toes to look great in my new sandals is very different from getting a pedicure because I realize I've exerted a lot of energy into caring for others this week, and treating myself to an experience where I can receive will refuel me so I can continue to give abundantly without feeling burnt out are two very different things. You see? A lot of times it's not what we're doing. It's the thought process, the intention, and the deeper meaning and understanding behind why we're doing it. Ideally, when you think about how you want to approach self-care you want balanced energy, wholeness, and nourishment to be at the forefront of your mind. Beauty, indulgence, and luxury can be extensions or byproducts of self-care, but they should not be motivating factors.

Practice. *Ideas include: Shutting the door at the office to put your legs up the wall and do a short guided meditation, spritz some lavender mist in the air, and read a positive article. Lock the bathroom door and take an epsom salt with lavender essential oil bubble bath. Scout out a local park to take a walk before you drop the kids off at school. Wake up before the rest of the house, enjoy a quiet cup of tea, and journal.*

"Taking good care of YOU means the people in your life will receive the best of you, rather than what's left of you."

—Carl Bryan

When I meet with clients and discuss self-care the most common statement I hear is similar to that when we discuss meditation, "I'd love to. I just don't have time." Years ago, my brother was obsessed with cars. During college, I would try to save money by only filling my tank a quarter or half way each time I went to the gas station. My brother explained to me that the car runs most efficiently on a full tank. He showed me how after the gas reaches the halfway mark it actually burns fuel faster and runs out of steam more quickly. He suggested I always top it off when I reach the half way mark. He explained how in the long run, that would actually save me money. Self-care works the same way. We are at our best and most efficient when our tank is full. It takes a lot more effort to get the same results when our tank is low. Practicing self-care is like topping off the fuel tank. It'll save us time and energy in the long haul. I know I said I rarely get sick, but recently I cashed in on one of my "rarely" moments; I was burning the candle at both ends. I was run down, but too stubborn to rest. My body whispered with fatigued, talked with exhaustion, and inevitable became ornery with my resistance to listen, so my body finally screamed. I got sick. In bed. No energy. No appetite. Just sleep. Sick. When I recovered just enough, I chose to carry on as though nothing happened. My sprightly Vata and ambitious Pitta dragged me out of bed; I convinced myself I could continue my work and activities as usual. By the end of the work week I was thoroughly depleted. Friday afternoon I was signing people into my yoga class and a student said, "How are you?" I finally admitted, "Tired." She asked if I had a busy week. I realized then, I hadn't done any more that week than a typical balanced week; the only difference was running on fumes required me to give 200% of my effort to reap at best, 50% of the results. I conceded to rest the entire weekend. We cannot afford a constant over expenditure of energy directed outwardly. We must redirect our flow of energy inwardly on a regular basis. Self-care is priceless.

Self-massage is the hallmark of self-care. Ayurveda recommends Abhyanga, or self-massage as a means to relax, restore, and rejuvenate. The word oil in Sanskrit is, Snehana. The word translates into English as love or affection. So every time you rub oil on the body you are applying love, and giving yourself affection. How sweet is that? The application of oil calms the nervous system, increases circulation, breaks up adipose tissue, flushes lymphatic congestion, sends toxins to the GI to be eliminated, hydrates the joints and nourishes the skin. You can lavish yourself with a daily massage in the morning before you shower or at night before you shower. Sesame oil is heating and should be used in the cooler months of the year because of the warming effects, and coconut oil is cooler and should be used during warmer times of year due to the cooling effects. Vatas are dry, so they should use more oil, and should use a firm and slow touch to feel grounded. Pittas are a little oily, so they should use a little less oil, and should use a deliberate touch to feel attended to. Pittas do well with starting their massage at the heart and allowing the hands and heat in the heart to radiate out. Using your hands smear the energy of the heart out—toward the lateral lines of the chest. This helps Pittas feel humble. Kaphas are should use the least amount of oil (as to avoid excess heaviness on the body), and should use a brisk touch to break up stagnation.Massaging head to toe is most grounding, while massaging the feet towards the head is more up-lifting. Apply the principles of opposites to create balance. If you feel energized, take advantage of grounding by massaging head to toe—guiding the energy down. If you feel fatigued, massage from the feet up to the head to lift your energy. You should do long strokes on the long bones, circles on the joints, and circles on the breasts and abdomen. Vatas, pay special attention to the hips and low back, as tension tends to gather there for you. Applying oil to the head not only feels great, it is calming for the mind and nervous system and nourishing for the hair. Moisturizing the scalp with oil even prevents premature graying and balding. Practice: Commit to giving yourself an oil massage this evening or tomorrow night. Take your time to touch, feel and celebrate your contours, texture and beautiful self.

> *"Self-compassion is simply giving the same kindness to ourselves that we would give to others."*
>
> **—Christopher Gerner**

There are a couple contraindications for Abhyanga. If there are a lot of toxins present in the GI tract then you would not want to give yourself a full body self—massage, because when there are too many toxins in the GI, the GI cannot digest the oil. Adding oil to toxicity will clog and congest the body. You will know if you have toxins in your GI by looking at your tongue. Go to the mirror and stick out your tongue. If you have a thick white or yellow coating on the tongue (especially near the back, that represents the colon), then you should not do Abhyanga on the entire body. You can drink ginger tea with a pinch of cinnamon once or twice a day until the coating on the tongue disappears.

Ginger tea with black pepper will help burn away the toxicity in the GI. Compliment these efforts by avoiding processed and heavy foods as your body is giving you the signal that your digestion has been compromised. You should also omit yourself from Abhyanga if you have had recent surgery, (you want to be cautious as to not infect wound), or if you have malignant tumors, (you do not want the massage to loosen and spread the imbalance). If this applies to you—you can concentrate your oil massage to a localized area like the feet or scalp. A head or foot massage feels amazing! There are dozens of tiny little Marma points, or energetic points on the head and feet. A massage is a great way to stimulate flow, loosen tension, and sink into relaxation. Note that when you want to wash the oil out of your hair, you should apply shampoo directly to the oily scalp before getting it wet. Massage the shampoo into the scalp, rinse, then shampoo and condition as usual.

People with a Kapha constitution or imbalance may forgo a self-massage for dry-brushing. Dry brushing helps stimulate circulation, break up adipose tissue, and drain stagnant lymph and fluid retention. This is best for Kapha. To dry brush, use a luffa brush or luffa gloves. With a bit of vigor brush towards your heart. Do long sweeps on that arms in the direction of the heart center, as well as up the legs towards the torso. Do this before you shower. Then if you'd like, you can massage a subtle layer of sesame oil over the body to soothe and nurture the skin and nervous system.

For Even Better Sleep...

Massage "Clarity" oil into the soles of the feet before bed. Take your time to really knead into arches to relieve unnecessary stress and tension. The blend of Sesame, Bhrami, Lavender, Eucalyptus and Lemon will calm your nervous system and restore your senses. (Clarity oil, by wellBlends…see references in the back of the book.)

> *"You'll never change your life until you change something you do daily. The secret of your success is found in your daily routine."*
>
> **—John C. Maxwell**

Dinacharya: Daily Routines: Bookend your day with routines. A morning routine will give you more energy and serve as a buffer for stresses that may surface later in the day. A nightly routine will help seal in a good day, erase the tension from a stressful day, help you sleep, and provide a freshener canvas for the new day ahead. Routines run in loops. Your routine should be as reliable as an invigorating sunrise, and as soothing as a melting sunset. To establish a routine is to establish a smart system you can rely on in times of ease and in times of stress. When you are stressed, cortisol and adrenaline cloud your thinking and impair your ability to make good decisions. A stable routine provides a stable dispensary of good choices. If we do not have a routine and we get stressed, we are likely to make poorer choices. It behooves us to have a routine that lessens our risk of making lousy choices in times of distress. Choices that are repeatedly made on a daily basis can be pre-made; this is the nature of a routine. Consistent. Positive. Supportive.

> *"Life is really simple, but we insist on making it complicated."*
>
> **—Confucius**

Morning Routines…By carving out time for yourself in the morning you will find yourself less reactive to hurdles throughout the day. Your morning sets the tone for your day. The law of attraction declares that we attract vibrations similar to our vibrations. Have you ever started out your day in a hurry and you find yourself hurried all day long? Have you ever woken up grouchy, started your day with one grouchy comment, and ended up riding the grouchy train all day? Hurried begets hurried. Grouchy begets grouchy. We can set the vibration we wish to see all day long by setting a Sankalpa, or an intention. Each morning, choose one or two words that embody the tone you'd like to experience that day. Perhaps your Sankalpa is, "I am energized. I am relaxed. I am abundant. I am forgiving. I am understood. I am adaptable. I am valued. I am helpful, or I am confident." There are no wrong intentions. If it comes from your heart—it is correct. State the intention in the morning and use that statement as a mental retreat when you need refuge throughout the day. In times when your day is free afflictions, you can reinforce this positive tone by repeating your Sankalpa when you feel grateful for your lovely day. Gratitude begets gratitude, and you will notice more items to be grateful for. A morning Sankalpa functions like the intention we set on our yoga mats at the start of the practice. Buddha said, "We are what we think. All that we are arises with our thoughts." There is no need to reserve such a powerful tool for our yoga practice exclusively, we can assimilate this tool into each day.

Sample Morning Routine:

» Wake up with the sunrise, or as close to it as possible to feed of the active solar energy for the day.

» Set your intention and repeat it several times.

» Eliminate to flush excess fluids, toxins and wastes from the body.

» Brush your teeth and scrape your tongue with a tongue scraper. A tongue scraper is a stainless steel U-shaped device that removes toxins from your tongue. Your tongue is a microcosm of your GI, so scraping your tongue removes toxins from the GI and stimulates strong digestion.

» Drink a glass of warm water water to flood out any residual toxicity. Drinking warm water is like giving your digestive system a shower.

» Meditate.

» Exercise—go for a walk, do yoga, or a few sun salutations. Stretch and get the Prana flowing.

» Give yourself a oil massage.

» Shower.

» Groom and dress for your liking.

» Eat a wholesome breakfast that compliments your Dosha.

Creating a daily routine may sound easy, but honor the distinction between simple and easy. Creating new habits requires diligence. As the saying goes, "Old habits die hard." Just because something is simple, doesn't mean it is easy. If this were easy, we would all be doing it already. Ayurveda refers to the idea of knowing what is best for you, and going against it anyway as Prajnaparadha. Prajnaparadha is, "A crime against wisdom." We commit

Prajnaparadha when we choose actions and behaviors knowing they are a detriment to our wellbeing. For example, I know crowding my schedule with too many back to back appointments can breed anxiety, but sometimes I do it anyway. I have friends who know drinking wine every night is contributing to their weight gain and fatigue, but they do it anyway. I am aware staying up too late, drinking too much coffee, skipping my morning practice, or answering emails at 9pm goes against my inner wisdom, but sometime I do it anyway. Beating ourselves up for not doing what we know we should will not improve our inner being. To avoid Prajnaparadha, set routines that provide support and make it easier to make positive decisions.

Get creative in customizing your routine…When my previous partner and I first moved in together we lived in a tiny studio apartment. We had to make compromise and figure out ways to make both of our morning routines feasible in such a small space. His morning routine to wake up, have coffee and breakfast, read the news on his I-pad, and have the news on in the background. This is how he grounded himself and fueled his energy for the day. I loved that he had a routine and wanted to be respectful of his sacred time. My routine was different. I liked to wake up, have coffee and a small bite to eat, and practice yoga to either in silence or to music. It only took a few days to notice that having the news on in the background created a negative shift in my tone for the day. For him, the news is just a source of information, he actually finds it relaxing. For me, starting my days with reports of murder and politics wasn't a soothing launchpad for the day. I find the news unnerving. It does not exemplify the language I want to replay all day. We agreed to have silence until the Today Show came on, (which tends to be slightly more upbeat than the local news). We both compromised to design a morning routine that honored our unique ways of minimizing stress and maximizing self-care.

> **Practice:** *Wake up with plenty of time to calibrate and declare your intention for the day. Give yourself time each morning for a self-massage to help protect you from stress and the threat of running out of fuel.*

The success of a good routine is in syncing up with the rhythms of nature. This includes following the natural tides of the sun and moon, not fighting the clock, and listening to your body. Ayurveda suggests that we go to bed and wake up around the same time each day. And eat our meals around the same time each day. Schedule time for activities that require energy by day, and time for resting and restoring by night. The sun's Yang energy is intrinsically active. We should wake up with the sun and borrow its active nature to move us through our day. The moon's Yin energy is inherently restorative. We should rest and repair with the moon's passive and rejuvenating energy.

> *"The motion of yin and yang generate all the things in nature."*
>
> **—Meh Juizhang & Guo Lei**

By eating our meals around the same time each day we will establish a rhythm. We are part of nature. By having a routine, we give our mind-body a sense that we are reliable stewards of our vessels. The structure doesn't need to be rigid or strict. There can be flexibly within the template. According to Ayurveda regular sleep and eating rhythms help boost our metabolism, productivity, and energy while alleviating stress and anxiety. There was a study where they interviewed American presidents. The question was, "How are you able to make such monumental decisions?" The presidents reported back with similar answers. The consensus was, they are able to make big decisions because the don't have to make little decisions. Their sleeping, eating and workout schedules have been arranged for them. Their clothes are out, and their food is ready. They do not have to consider small decisions like, "Hmmm should I hit snooze or get up now?" "Should I work through lunch and leave early or run and grab something now?" "Hmmm should I have the chicken wrap or humus plate?" "Should I go to yoga class or the gym?" Nope. They don't have to weigh the pros and cons of any of these common choices. The minutiae of decision making can breed indecision, uneasiness, and pressure. Presidents alleviate themselves from small decisions so they have the brain space to make big decisions. Sure, no one is going to lay out our clothes, make all our meals, and schedule our personal training sessions, but we can replicate a similar concept in our own lives. With a little planning, we can design a structure according to our Dosha and lifestyle that will free us up to live more freely. All humans do well with routines. Look at kids, they need routine and structure. They flourish with regular school times, designated recess, and weekends off. (Kids who are home schooled also have a sense of structure and reliability.) These predictable patterns make kids feel safe and provided for. This is true for adults as well. Even patterns like consistent paychecks, or simple pleasures like our favorite weekly TV show and yoga class provide us with a sense of stability.

Routines are helpful for everyone, but glaringly important for Vata Dosha because Vatas have a tendency to fly by the seat of their pants. People with a Vata imbalance will not instinctually create order, but once they establish into a routine, they will feel much better. Vata types who are in balance, have already realized they need a routine to feel safe and content in the world. It is material that a Vata's routine gives space for freedom. We do not want our little Vata to feel like a caged bird. Pittas tend to instinctively create routines for the sake of productivity and efficiency. Kaphas are go with the flow and will follow along with a given routine without a fight (Unless of course that routine requires them to get up too early or move too fast). As you come into balance you may notice the areas where you gravitate and feel inclined to spend extra time. Vata types may need more time in prayer or meditation to ground. Pitta types may need a bit longer with a sweet and cooling coconut oil massage. Kapha types may recognize that they need to get up earlier and make morning movement a priority. We will never fit into neatly groomed one size fits all boxes. The specifics of our approach and routines will need to be tailored to fit the uniqueness of our lives.

Throughout the Day: Here we will identify the brush stroke principles that help any combination of Doshas stay in balance. Generally, we're talking about an organic blend of avoiding extremes and respecting natural urges.

» Avoid harsh environments like too much sun, heat, rain, cold and wind. Any extreme condition (especially unexpected and prolonged conditions) will start to tamper with your elemental make up. You learned this when you were little and your mom said, "Don't go outside with wet hair when it's cold. You'll get a cold."

» Pace yourself. Try not to overload your schedule or datebook things in a way that creates a feeling of being rushed. This is significant for Vata types and people with Vata imbalances. Pittas you can manage a packed schedule, but that doesn't mean you should routinely do it. The stress can raise your cortisol, heat, and agitation levels. Err on the side of caution—pace yourself.

» Don't suppress your natural urges. Coughing, laughing, eliminating, passing gas, the urge to vomit, crying, and ejaculating are all natural urges. Suppressing natural urges can create an imbalance. It is a natural urge to sweat. No one goes to the gym, gets hot and looks down at their pores and thinks, "Please don't sweat. please don't sweat. please don't sweat." But I mustn't be alone in eating something that didn't agree with me, feeling my belly churn, clenching my buttocks and thinking, "Please don't toot. please don't toot." I realize we have cultural etiquette around our behaviors, but it's worth noting that suppressing urges on a regular basis will create more chronic imbalances. There are parts of the world where spitting and belching are welcomed. I'm not suggesting we turn the table on cultural etiquette, but we can surely press the borders where being polite and protecting our health collide.

» Protect your sense organs. Wear sunglasses when the sun is shining brightly. Try to avoid too much time in front of the computer, smartphone, or television. Avoid loud noises like a lot of construction or an abundance of concerts. The eyes, ears, nose, skin and tongue and incredibly valuable. Protect them. Try not to overuse them. According to Ayurveda, one of the leading causes of disease is the overuse or misuse of the sense organs. (Watching or listening to programs with violent or negative messages falls into the category of misusing sense organs.)

"Look deep into nature and then you will understand everything better."

—Albert Einstein

Seal your day with serenity. Embedded in the tides of life, it is written within the laws of nature that all things come and go. Sunrise and sunsets provide a daily reminder to the impermanence of conditions, and the ability to refresh and begin anew. An evening routine will help you rinse away the tensions of a tough day, and seal in the flavors of a good day. An evening self-care routine will help you sleep and feel refreshed in the morning.

Sample Evening Routine:

- Eat a light dinner
- Go for a evening walk
- Give yourself an oil massage
- Take a warm shower
- Drink Golden Milk or chamomile tea
- Unplug from computers, social media, the TV and phone
- Read a book or write in your journal
- Fall asleep to a Yoga Nidra, meaning yogic sleep guided meditation

Spend time in nature. Nature is medicinal. Spending time in nature or even just viewing scenes of nature reduces stress, releases fear, provokes optimism, reduces your blood pressure, alleviates muscle tension and regulates your heart rate. Being engrossed in nature helps us cope with pain because nature is a healing distraction from aches and discomforts that may otherwise occupy our attention. There was a recent study of patients who underwent gallbladder surgery. In the recovery rooms half of the patients had a view of trees, the others had a view of a blank wall. The findings revealed that the patients who had the view of the trees tolerated pain better and experienced faster healing processes. Spending time in nature is enlightening. You never see a depressed bunny, a flower that's hurrying to grow, a cloud that's too attached to release its rain, or a lightning bolt that's too inhibited to reveal its passion. I've never seen an eager pond or a competitive butterfly. Nature has a way of restoring sanity and bringing peace through its patient and humble ways. Nature has a way of reversing adverse emotions. Due to nature's inherently pleasing and interesting aesthetics, nature is proven to help increase our ability to pay attention. When we are in nature we intuitively focus on what we are experiencing. In recent studies, it has been shown that children with ADHD, (a Vata imbalance) who spend time in nature have higher attention spans. Nature is a safe haven even if there is a little payment involved. Get outside. If the midday heat is too much, (especially for Pitta Dosha), try a revitalizing sunrise stroll or meander in the residual goodness of a lingering sunset. Feel the grass under your feet, let your fingers skim the water, have lunch under a tree, bring flowers into your home. The options are endless. There is a whole world beyond the interstate and iPhone. As often as you can, get outside, bring the outside in, get to know nature.

Hiccups in routine & one's ability to adapt…Becoming a mom to a puppy threw me through a loop. Clearly my naivety lead me to believe being responsible for a living being would seamlessly blend into my life. False. I experienced a rocky adjustment period upon adopting a puppy. Due to my propensity to become Vata imbalanced, I am a creature of habit. I tether myself to daily routines as to not feel like a butterfly on amphetamines. I should call my puppy my guru, because they say you learn the most from the things that challenge you. My puppy is my teacher. While I consider myself nurturing, my pup revealed my ostensibly selfish traits. There's nothing like a living creature who depends on you to derail your pockets of peace and copious hours of alone time. I quickly realized that while routines help us stay grounded, our happiness is not composed of a neatly-micromanaged profile of routines. Routines must be malleable to the flow of life. Happiness is an extension of the ability to adapt and respond to the fluctuations of life. I applied an idiom I learned years back, "What you do does not matter most. What you are thinking while you are doing it matters more." I reframed my thoughts to transform taking my puppy out at 3am. I reshaped my thoughts from being annoyed to being caring while picking up toys and cleaning up accidents during what used to be pockets of downtime. I began incorporating my breathing practices into our middle of the night tinkle session and repeated daily affirmations on our morning walks.

PAUSE FOR AFFIRMATION

"I am devoted to taking care of myself."

Essential Oils for the Doshas… Vatas do well with warming, sweet, and calming essential oils such as: lavender, cinnamon, nutmeg, chamomile, ylang ylang, and frankincense. Pittas do well with cooling oils such as: fennel, sandalwood, peppermint, and lemongrass. And Kaphas do best with invigorating oils such as: eucalyptus, rosemary, peppermint, and basil. To use oils, you can add 6-8 drops to your bath. You can diffuse the oils into the air at home or work, or you can apply a drop to your wrist and behind your ear.

"Adopt the pace of nature. Her secret is patience."

—Ralph Waldo Emerson

Mama Points and Face Massage..."Don't touch your face!" This statement blared through chambers of my mind anytime my hands crept up to access, rub, or god forbid, "pick at" my face. I was blessed and cursed with extreme adult onset acne. I say blessed because a) when traditional dermatological approaches didn't stick, my blemish dilemmas inspired me to learn more about natural health b) handed me a lesson in compassion and empathy c) gave me an "in your face" lesson on how our thoughts and emotions manifest physically. I learned that what we eat can sabotage our skin. Wholefoods heal, whereas excess salt, caffeine, acids, and chemicals reck havoc on our skin. I learned to be kind to myself when I looked in the mirror. I had to cultivate compassion towards myself and truthful understand that my beauty and worth had nothing to do with my reflection. This awakening gave me empathy towards others struggling with their own hardships; however big or small they may be. And finally, I learned that our skin is symbolic of how we see ourselves. If we see ourselves as flawed humans, this can manifest as flawed skin. If we're angry, our skin can look angry and inflamed. Everything physical has a corresponding mental/ emotional counter part. Our skin has a lot to teach us.

As a young adult two key lessons were drilled into my mind: stay away from oil and all oil based products and never touch your face. This advice couldn't have been more backwards. Oils actually offer our skin support. Oils like coconut and almond are anti-inflammatory. Oils like neem and tea tree are anti-fungal and anti-microbial. Oils like lavender and frankincense calm irritated skin (and emotions). Quality, organic oils in general are nutrient rich and nurturing. Lathering ourselves in oil is easy way to practice self-care. Ayurveda teaches us that self-care is one of the most accessible ways to establish and maintain our highest states of wellbeing. A facial abhyanga, or facial massage is an easy way to give yourself some love!

Try this:

Take one teaspoon of coconut oil. 2 drops of tea tree, 2 drops of lavender, and one drop of frankincense. Stir the oils together in a small dish. Wash your face with warm water and a gentle scrub. Using your hands, smear the botanical oils onto your face. Massage in large circles over the entire face, smaller circles on the cheeks, and even smaller circles around the eyes. From the center of your brow across the length of the forehead use your pointer and middle fingers to brush upwards strokes. Repeat this three times. Then take a small amount of oil and brush from the collar bone up towards your chin. Repeat this three times. Use your pointer finger and thumb to trace along the jaw bone. Massage gently to relieve stress and pressure stored in the jaw. (This helps alleviate TMJ and stress headaches).

When your finished you'll feel and look radiant. You can sleep in the oils or splash warm water in your face and gently pat a towel on your moisturized and cared for skin.

To take it one step further, you can press on your "Marma", or acupuncture points. Each point correlates with a particular physical and mental aspect of your mind/body. These points help us balance our energy, lymphatic, nervous, and circulatory systems. Use your middle fingers and apply a moderate amount of pressure for 30 seconds to one minute.

1. Centre of the chin (reproductive region)
2. The corners of the mouth (metabolism)
3. Between nose and upper lip (cerebral circulation)
4. The outer corners of the nose (sinuses)
5. Centre of cheekbones (lungs)
6. Lower lids, just above the cheekbones (adrenals)
7. Junction between eyebrows and nose, on the lower part of the eyebrow ridge (liver/spleen)
8. Temples (stress headaches and colon)
9. Third eye (6th chakra)
10. Crown of the head: place hands on crown of head and massage with your finger pads (crown chakra)

This therapeutic treatment is not about vanity. Real self-care is about nourishment on the levels of understanding, compassion, and balance for all three bodies: physical, mental, and emotional. Enjoy your beautiful self and this therapeutic recipe for inner and outer beauty.

CHAPTER NINE

Healthy Bowels

"The road to good health is paved with good intestines."

—Sherry A. Rogers

"Not to cleanse the colon is like having the entire garbage collecting staff in your city go on strike for days end. The accumulation of garbage in the street creates putrid, odoriferous, unhealthy gases which are dispersed into the atmosphere."

—Dr. Norman Walker

TAKING CARE OF Your Bowels: Duty calls. Healthy elimination could be the key to your health. No one wants to talk about it, in fact I had a challenging time trying to figure out where I could eloquently slip it into this book. So I didn't. Here it is. I'm immune to what some might deem awkward when it comes to discussing fecal matter. Our elimination can tell us a lot about our health. In such, I always ask my clients, "How is your elimination?" Nine times out of ten, the client turns pink and quickly and quietly says, "Normal." Your bowels and the removal of waste through proper excretions are critical to your health. According to Ayurveda, 80% of disease originate it the digestive tract. "Normal" is too vague. Let's discuss details.

3 things that matter when it comes to digestion and elimination:

1. What we eat.
2. How we break it down and assimilate it.
3. How we get rid of the waste.

Digestion, assimilation and elimination are crucial to longevity. We consume sights, sounds, smells, thoughts and experiences, everything we consume must be digested, absorbed, and eliminated in due time. Everything we consume throughout out human experience effects us, but food has a special physical significance because the substances we eat form building blocks for creating, sustaining, or destroying our bodies. We need high quality, nutrient rich foods to protect our high quality, nutrient rich bodies. Food stuff is broken down through an astute process in an area known as the GI tract, or digestive tract. Food must be broken down into smaller molecules to be absorbed by the blood and carried throughout the body. The GI includes the esophagus, stomach, small intestine, large intestine, pancreas, liver and gallbladder. We have the capability to renew energy, grow, and repair cells thanks to these organs and processes. While the

Pitta is the queen of transformation and metabolism, all three Doshas have their hand in the digestive process. The water quality of Kapha helps us break down food in the mouth by utilizing our saliva secretions.The nose is the sense organ of Kapha. When we breathe in the aroma of appetizing food we create more saliva secretions in excited anticipation for the meal to come. Food that is pleasing to your senses physiologically aids in your ability to digest it. The movement quality of Vata steps in to helps us to swallow and transport the food, brining it down the esophagus and into the stomach. It important to slow down and chew thoroughly so that Vata's speedy nature does not succeed in rushing large pieces of food down the pipes. Large pieces of food are harder to break down and depress timely elimination. Next, Pitta steps in secreting digestive juices, enzymes and acids within the stomach, liver, pancreas, and gallbladder that help to covert big molecules into smaller more useable molecules. The strength of your digestive juices is directly related to the strength of your Agni, or digestive fire. We want to keep this zone incandescent. The small intestine completes the breakdown process, then absorbs most of the digested food, water and minerals passing them along to other parts of the body for storage and further conversions. Consuming pure, high quality foods assures that we will absorb the best of the best. It would be a cruel challenge to expect the body to convert junk into greatness. So what we eat is a huge factor in optimum assimilation. The final part of the process is to eliminate the unused or useless food remains. If we don't get rid of the waste, the waste festers and turns toxic in our bodies. We call these toxins, AMA which means undigested thoughts, emotions, experiences—and in this case, food. Toxins in the bowels don't stay in the bowels. The toxins can float into the blood, and surface to the skin as acne or rashes. Toxins find their way into joint cavities creating inflammation and arthritis, or sit in the intestines creating obstructions, bloating and flatulence. Idle toxins can even stop the downward flow of energy. This stagnation and impediment can breed anxiety, irritation and depression.

> *"If the sewer system in your home is backed up, your entire home is affected. Should it be any different in your body?"*
>
> **—Norman Walker DSc.**

The term,"Regular" in reference to bowel movements varies from person to person. Generally less than 3 movements in a week means your bowels are sluggish, and more than 3 in a day means your bowels are hyper. Ideally, we want our stools to be formed into the shape of a capital letter J. The stool should be smooth and easy to pass. Stools that are dry and pellet like or require pushing are indicative of cold, rough, and dry conditions that are consistent with a Vata imbalance.

6 Ways to way to promote proper elimination:

1. Eat more roughage. Cooked roughage is easier to breakdown and smoother to pass. Raw and cold foods require the heated atmosphere of our digestive fire to do all the work. When we cook food we initiate the release of active enzymes and alleviate our bodies from facilitating 100% of the conversion. Cooking roughage like spinach, kale, mustard greens, dandelion greens, and calciferous vegetables like broccoli and cauliflower also helps release the water content that is locked into the vegetables. Cooking converts the texture from dry and

hard to moist and soft. Moist and soft is easier to assimilate and pass. Avoid overcooking veggies as to retain nutrients. You want the vegetable to keep its coloring and a hint of crunch to assure you have retained the nutritional value. Burnt veggies are devoid of nutrients because at that point you've cooked out all the Prana. Think of it in terms of sunbathing. Thirty minutes in the sun gives you a nice warm glow and enhances your vitality, a whole day in the direct sun leaves you charred and energetically wiped out. We want the warm glow and vitality version of cooking. Sauté, stir-fry, bake, roast and simmer. Do not burn.

2. Use healthy oils like olive oil, coconut oil, grapes oil, and ghee in foods to create lubrication. There are approximately 25 feet from the mouth to the anus. If the channels are dry and rough particles get stuck. Stuck particles stagnate into toxic buildup. Lubricated pipes are essential for good plumbing. Vata types tend to be exceptionally dry, so Vatas should take care to use plenty of oil to moisturize their elimination channels. In addition to lubrication, vitamins A,D,E and K are fat soluble, meaning they will not dissolve without the presence of fat. Good fats function as excellent vehicles for driving essential nutrients into the tissues. Olive oil should not get too hot. You can drizzle olive oil on salads, roasted vegetables (after cooking) and grains. Coconut oil, grape seed oil, and ghee are excellent cooking agents. I use these oils for sautéing and baking. You can also add a generous dab to soups, grains and roasted vegetables. For example, I'll have a teaspoon of ghee in oatmeal with a dash of cinnamon—or a tsp of coconut oil on a sweet potato with a pinch of cardamom.

3. Drink more water. It would be tricky to wash your car without water. It is just as tricky to wash your intestines without water. Water should be the staple fluid in your world. Sometimes we think we're drinking enough but we need to keep in mind that not all fluids are hydrating. Coffee, soda and other caffeinated beverages cause more frequent urination and promote dehydration. Fruit juices that are high in electrolyte and mineral potassium serve as a diuretic as well. Pineapple and citrus juices have their benefits, but they are not hydrating. And sorry gals, alcohol doesn't count either. Recently, I had a client complain of constipation. When I inquired about her fluid intake she told me she drinks, "plenty". She said it with a cute confident smile. She was so confident I nearly just moved on to deeper inquiries, but something told me to ask her to elaborate. I asked her specifically as to what she drinks. She told me she has two cups of coffee in the morning, a diet coke at work, green tea on the way to the gym, a glass of water with dinner and a glass of wine before bed. She was correct. She was drinking, but with the exception of her water with dinner, all of her fluids were diuretics that were actually drying her out. She made a few adjustments by adding a glass of warm water in the morning, drinking her two cups of coffee and then switching to warm water with lemon in the afternoon and evening and a mug of golden milk to replace her wine before bed. She reported back that her bowels became normal, and she enthusiastically added in that her wrinkles diminished. I smiled and explained that wrinkles are the result of dryness. We must stay hydrated from the inside out to maintain that dewy glow. Exact water needs vary based on a person's size, environment

and activity level. Nothing about taking care of ourselves is exact for everyone across the board. We're simply different from one another. Generally, people who live in arid climates like the desert and people with very slight builds and crackly joints, (Vata) require even more water to counterbalance the abundance of dryness. Pittas and athletes tend to need more water because the sweat more. It's important to replenish lost fluids. In the summer, everyone sweats more, so we should all drink more. Even though it may be hot outside, remember not to douce your GI with ice cold water because that sort of extreme will create an imbalance and completely extinguish your digestive fire. In the summer, room temperature water is perfect. Due to Kaphas tendency to hold onto things, water included, they require less than their Vata and Pitta friends, but should still take care to stay hydrated. If you wait until you are thirsty to drink, you are already dehydrated. Generally, drinking about 8 glasses of warm or room temperature water a day is a good baseline. Remember to start your day with warm water to nudge motility. Drinking warm water after brushing your teeth and scraping your tongue will help flush residual toxins out of the body. It is important to note, that there IS such thing as drinking too much water. Drinking too much can tax your kidneys and dilute your digestive fire. Balance requires moderation. Too much of anything can create an imbalance—water included.

4. Remove dairy and red meat. Heavy animal products are difficult to process and delay transient time. A vegetarian meal takes on average 27-61 hours to digest and exit, whereas a non-veg meal can take up to 96 hours to

breakdown and pass. Dairy and red meat are the hardest to break down. They create cellular inflammation and congestion that cause the intestinal lining to swell. Essentially everything gets puffy, slow, and irritated. Puffy, slow, and irritated are not the kind of qualities that drive movement. Lighter foods such as plant based foods digest faster and easier than animal products.

5. Eat more fiber. Fiber gets things moving! Soluble fiber attracts water and helps create a gel like bind. Apples, beans, oats, and flaxseeds are great sources. Insoluble fiber can not be broken down, so it acts like a broom sweeping through the GI grabbing food and speeding it along. Great sources include broccoli, whole grains, nuts, leafy greens and grapes. We can get all the fiber we need from a balanced diet of vegetables, fruits, whole grains, beans, legumes, nuts and seeds. A perfect example of a daily meal plan with adequate fiber would be, quinoa with baked apples and cinnamon and ghee for breakfast. A sweet potato with flaxseed and coconut oil with sautéed broccoli drizzled in olive oil for lunch, a few nuts of fresh fruit as a snack and a broth based bean soup for dinner.

6. Elimination is a movement. Movement propels movement. Exercise, move your body, stretch, twist, walk, jump, swim, and dance. Get creative. It doesn't have to be a formal workout. Exercise accelerates your breathing and heart rate. This helps to stimulate the natural contraction of intestinal muscles. Muscle contractions expedite the elimination process. Yoga moves like bending and twisting help to free up space for the digestive organs, while stimulating peristalsis. Get moving to get things moving.

Other Factors:

Physiological Factors: Psychological factors can urge or impair peristalsis. Stress and anxiety can exacerbate faulty plumbing. Fear is an emotion of constriction. Constipation is an imbalance of constriction. Allowing yourself to literally, "Let go" is beneficial. Bowel movements are associated with the first Chakra, the area of survival, security and stability. As we learned earlier, if you feel insecure in regard to your basic needs being met because your concerned about your finances or safety your first Chakra may be weakened. A closed first Chakra depresses the ability to eliminate. You can try the Chakra meditation to open that area and revive natural functions. Sitting on the ground in nature will help root you. That feeling of being rooted with nurture your first Chakra. You'll recall that every experience expresses itself in the body. Seek out experiences that help you flow, release, and let go. Dancing, painting, or purging old clutter can all help you learn to let go.

> **Practice—**Root Chakra Meditation: *Sit on the ground and repeat this affirmation, "I am connected to all that is around me. This connection gives me a strong foundation and does not hold me back. Security and stability in life allow me to move with both confidence and connection to who I am. I trust that I am safe. I am willing to let go."*

Patterns: What goes in must come out. Eating breakfast, lunch, and dinner around the same time each day will generate a more patterned evacuation schedule. Your body will come to know your rhythm and will begin to synchronize with it. Feast or famine creates confusion. If the body doesn't know when it'll receive its next meal, it is less likely to quickly burn and eliminate excess; it is fearful that it will not receive more. It is kind of like your spending habits. You are more likely to spend your money freely if you are used to getting a paycheck on a regular basis. You would be less likely to spend freely if you have no clue as to when you would get paid again. The body is logical in that way. Become regular in your eating patterns to become regular in your elimination patterns.

Traveling: Many people suffer from constipation while traveling. The speed and movement involved in traveling can dry us out. Think of the movement of fan blades, it creates a drying effect. Traveling exacerbates Vata, and constipation is a condition of heightened Vata. Flying is especially Vata exasperating because of the speed and high altitudes involved in the mode of transportation. Traveling can also place us in unfamiliar environments and take us away from our usual and comfortable patterns. All of these factors increase Vata. Taking special care to pacify Vata while traveling is important. Try a grounding oil massage once you arrive at your destination. Also try to keep your routine of regular mealtimes and incorporate plenty of warm, moist, and fiber rich foods when you are away from home. Drink extra warm water to counterbalance the drying effects of travel. You can even add a teaspoon of ghee to hot water to hydrate and lubricate at the same time. I find that if i'm backed up while traveling, a hot bath, a warm mea,l and glass of hot water with ghee before bed usually does the trick.

Avoid Laxatives. Over the counter laxatives create dependency. The colon gradually loses its tone and becomes lazy. Abusing laxatives can create electrolyte and mineral deficiencies. The body is a wellspring of immutable alchemy. When we routinely give the body a crutch like a laxative, our natural functions begin to weaken or atrophy. An all natural herb called, Triphala is a wonderful substitute to laxatives. This plant medicine will help gather toxins, guide them to the intestines, bulk stools, and promote evacuation in most people's. Take it before bed with a cup of warm water. Triphala can be taken for prologued periods of time and will not create dependency. See a practitioner to guarantee safe usage and results. Senna leaf is another gentle laxative. It comes in a tea format. I would reserve the tea for traveling or once a week usage at most. If you suffer from chronic constipation at home, in addition to everything above—incorporate aloe vera gel into your nightly routine. One or two tablespoons at night will serve as a gentle laxative. Drinking Golden Milk before bed is another way to calm the nervous system, reduce inflammation in the colon, and relax so that you can release, shall we say.

A Tasty Way to Alleviate Constipation…If you drink coffee, add 1 teaspoon of Golden Milk powder to your morning brew, along with 1 teaspoon of coconut oil. The coffee works to expedite motility and the oil helps to lubricate your internal channels. The ingredients in Golden Milk help assist in proper digestion:

» ginger—stokes Agni.

» turmeric—reduces inflammation in the colon.

» nutmeg—calms the nervous system, so the bowels are not tense.

» cinnamon—promotes increased circulation and general flow of movement.

» cardamom—relieves indigestion that contributes to occasional back-ups.

The addition of coconut oil is essential because the vitamins and integral properties in Golden Milk are fat soluble. The ingredients will not assimilate in plain coffee or even hot water. The added bonus is—it tastes amazing! If you have a severe Vata or Pitta imbalance, coffee is not recommended because it's too stimulating and heating.

PART II

Nutriton and Healing

"There is no diet that will do what healthy eating does. Skip the diet. Just eat healthily."

—Anonymous

NUTRITION PREFACE

HUNGER IS NOT always about food. Nourishment is not always about vitamins and minerals. We have an appetite for life and a desire to be nourished physically, mentally and emotionally. Sometimes we have to ask the questions—What am I really hungry for? What satisfies me? Am I full? Have I been consuming what is best for me? These questions are not exclusive to our pallet and gut. These questions prompt us to lovingly and correctly fill our plates, our lives, and our souls. I think it is fair to presume that diet, nutrition, and body image are near—and possibly uncomfortably dear to all of us. Our relationship with ourselves, and our relationship with food are two of the most intimate relationships we possible have in our lifetime. The sanctity of these relationships should be caressed with acceptance, self-love, and appreciation. I'd like to share a short story that is a prologue to the story at the start of the book. I love stories because we all have our own authentic script, but within the uniqueness of each personal story, we meet together, with shared themes that penetrate the most sincere places in all of our lives.

"We all feel the same. Just a different times."

—Kathryn Budig

As a kid I ran around in my little body impervious to the ideas of sickness or health. As a teenager I was confused by my rapidly changing body. It seemed to morph faster than I could keep up with. Ill equipped with an understanding of my mind, body, and soul—nor the appropriate tools to manage my evolving self. I became frustrated, overwhelmed, and abusive towards myself. I spent an entire year living on primarily grapes and tiny handfuls of cereal. I was diagnosed with anorexia nervosa. I had developed a fearful relationship with food and how it would influence me. I pounded my fragile joints running on a treadmill for hours on end, watching calories burn. Irrespective of the way I looked. I hated my body. I later realized eating disorders have very little to do with, "The way we look". I popped laxatives like candy and isolated myself from what was previously, my happy little world. I distanced myself from my friends, the activities I loved, and everything that made me smile—all because I was gravely confused and misinformed on how to accept, love, and take care of myself. Disheartened by the negative attention of concerned parents, teachers, and friends I conceded to my parents wishes for me to go to nutritionists, counselors, and psychologists. A typical counseling or psychiatric appointment consisted of me sitting in a cold doctors office shivering with my arms crossed over my waist. My vacant eyes dazed off as I listened just enough to follow through on what they expected of me. However, there was one nutritionist who was immensely helpful. She spoke to me like a person, not a disease. She gave me practical ideas and small benchmark goals that seemed safe and achievable. My turnaround gained momentum when I overheard a conversation between my mom and step-dad. I was walking downstairs when I heard them contemplating refinancing the house and working out strategies to pay for my expensive, "In-patient care". That same week I meandered out of a doctors where they were checking my heart (my weight had dropped so low it was taxing my heart) to see my mom, dad and step-dad waiting for me. To have them all there in one room made their concern and the severity of the situation glaringly obvious to me. I knew then, something had to change. I then took what I then knew to be the appropriate steps to climb out of the sad and self-destructive pit. Physically, I gained weight and looked more, "Normal", but mentally and emotionally I was still severely disconnected from my True Nature. During the last few years of my high school career I flipped to completely neglecting my body. I ate whatever junk it is teenagers nonchalantly eat, I got wrapped up in boyfriends, experimenting with drugs, and teenage dramas. I am clearly not proud of those experiences. I wouldn't recommend that painful route to anyone. The reason I share these experiences is because now, decades later, I see the silver lining. I am grateful for the dark days and even my horrible decisions, because they brought me to where I am now. I know my passion to uncover truths and tools, my relentless mission to share the principles I practice and speak about, as well as my wholehearted pursuit to help others was born from those trying times. I do not share this for attention, sympathy, or response. Our suffering cannot be compared to another's suffering. We all experience our own unique magnitude of human emotions. We travel along the shared spectrum of human emotions through different experiences. But, I am grateful, and do consider myself blessed and fortunate. The pain I inflicted was always in my control. On some subconscious level, I was pulling my own puppet strings. Fortunately, I was surrounded by love. Love makes all the difference. It is my hope that everyone who collapses into periods of pain, can be quickly scooped up by arms of love. If not others, than the drawing forth of your own. I see the value in adversity, because I know the hues of this life give us texture, dimension, empathy and strength.

In college I more or less just let my body be. I wasn't purposefully destructive or healing. It wasn't until after college that I began to travel. When I moved to China, I ate the local fresh cuisine, I rode my bike down to the Yu-Long river, and read books every afternoon. I took yoga classes after enjoyable days of teaching English at a vocational college in stunning Yangshou, China. It was starting to dawn on me that lifestyle plays a fundamentally important role in feeling good. On the most subtle of levels, I was starting to get it. It wasn't until I dove into yoga and Ayurveda that I began to feel the way I thought I should have been feeling all along. I was finally given the tools and the language to comprehend everything I already intuitively knew. I started to dismantle the lies media and advertising would love us to believe. I gave up diet crap, I started to eat real food, exercise because I wanted to, not because I had to, unwind, and finally sleep well. For the fist time in nearly ten years, I stopped trying to fix my body, ignore it, or outsmart it. I finally started to understand it. I retrieved my sense of admiration and respect for my healthy arms that could give hugs, eyes that could see clearly, strong jaw that could chew, and resilient heart that would carry me through vigorous workouts and the loss of people I love. I finally gained an appreciation for the powerful, miraculous, and beautiful vessel—the human body. Everyday I find myself excited to learn more, practice my learnings, and share fervently. Not because I want everyone to live this exact way, not because I think this is the only "right" way, but because if I knew what I know now, I could have saved myself a lot of suffering. While those lessons were necessary and valuable, I have full faith in these teachings.

"The lotus flower blooms beautifully from the deepest and thickest mud."

—Buddhist Proverb

CHAPTER TEN

Debunking Modern Myths

"Eat food. Mostly plants. Not too much."

—Michael Pollan

FOOD NOT ONLY feeds our bodies, it fuels our spirits. Never put your spirit on a diet. I grew up in a home where love was unconditional, but food was the host for conditions. Foods with fat made you fat, and diet foods promised you thinness. I trusted the numbers on plastic and foil wrappers more than I trusted the instinctual cues from my body. My eating was calculated. God willing, if I ate the recommended amount of carbs, sugars, calories, proteins, and fats maybe I would get to bask in the phantom world where skinny rests beautifully alongside happiness and fields of dandelions. Funny truth about this approach—constantly monitoring my food made me obsess about food. This obsession distorted my relationship with food, my body, and my confidence into a conditional heaven or hell determined by the numbers on labels and the numbers on a scale. My tumultuous relationship with food was paved from a place of believing the destructive lie—that I was not enough. So much of what you are reading is the positive reverberation of realizing, I am enough. But, what I knew about nourishment was not enough. I decided then, it was my quest to debunk the disorienting lies around food. It was my mission to understand nourishment on every level. I approached the pursuit with this in mind—A nutrition label would not suffice to nourish me. I was determined to find out what would. What really fills us up? What makes us feel energized? What are the proper building blocks for strong bones and rich blood? I am no wise sage. I am a woman who appreciates vitality. I crave vivid colors, creativity, purity, and substance. To taste these qualities in life—taste them in your food. I shun the idea of being labeled and judged, put me in a box and eventually I will feel restricted and depleted. If I do not want to be labeled and boxed up, why would I eat food that is? Choosing what food works best for us is not a matter of arithmetic. It is a matter of nature, liveliness, and intuition. Food not only feeds our bodies, it fuels our spirits. Never put your spirit on a diet.

> *"The food you eat can be either the safest and most powerful form of medicine, or slowest form of poison."*
>
> **—Ann Wigmore**

Ayurveda speaks to nutrition from the vantage point of nature, qualities, and tastes. Ayurvedic nutrition is enlightening and healing, but before we get there we have to stop the bleeding. I had a client come in for a follow-up and she said, "Kristen, I was looking over the packet you gave me and I saw I that zucchini is not good for me because I have a Kapha imbalance. Should I really never eat zucchini?" I had to tell her, "You expressed that you currently grab fast food for lunch everyday and eat microwave meals for dinner. Eating more of any vegetable would be an improvement. For now, do not worry about the details. Eat more vegetables. You have a green light to eat as much of and as many types of vegetables as you want. Free of analysis and restraint, eat your veggies." I am not speaking from a pedestal here. I can relate. I have absolutely no judgement. I did the same thing for years. Quick, easy, convenient, and denatured food is our cultural norm. But, just because much our culture has morphed into accepting a damaging sense of normal, does not mean the choices we make should accept or enable the harmful trend. Prior to absorbing what is best for us, we should examine and unleash ourselves from the myths and misunderstandings that misguide and limit us. Food is such an integral part of all of our lives. We are each enter conversations about food with a deeply personal catalog of preexisting information, beliefs, and ideals. Nutrition is not a new topic for you. We are bombarded with nutrition claims, fads, and "groundbreaking reports" on a daily basis. Yet, truly understanding nutrition remains elusive to must of us. Recognizing where we originated, where we currently are, and where we want to go in regard to food, food culture, and food facts will help illuminate our path. Ayurveda was realized over 5,000 years ago. I am willing to bet that the food system of millenniums ago would hardly recognize the food system of today. The way our food is grown, sourced, packaged, distributed, and consumed is a world away from where is was over 5,000 years ago. Food and "food stuff" is alien as compared to even as recent as fifty years ago. Do you think your grandmother knows what a 'go-gurt' is? What about a zone bar, hot pockets, or Monster? Probably not. We live in a quick moving world, accompanied by rapidly changing thoughts and beliefs. Each of our individual ideologies about food drives the enormously personal choices we make when it comes to our nourishment, or lack thereof. Let us cleanse ourselves from popular fallacies so we can make informed and honest choices.

> *"A wise person is hungry for knowledge, while a fool feeds on trash."*
>
> **—Anonymous**

Misconceptions…

Calorie Counting is a Flawed Approach. Not all calories are created equal. There are 100 calories in a large organic apple and 100 calories in a snack bag of Cheetos. Do you think these two sources of calories are equivalent? No. The nutrient to calorie ratio is completely different. An apple is loaded with vitamins, fiber, and antioxidants. An apple is loaded with Prana, while Cheetos are lacking Prana, they are actually depleting your bank of nutrients. Food that is devoid of Prana is devoid of energetic and nutritional value. Advertisements crack me up. I love the one where the two girls return home from the gym and one of the girls opens the refrigerator and grabs a canister of spray of whipped cream from the fridge and starts squirting it into her mouth. The other girl is collapsed on the floor from the bliss of her work out. She says, "What?! Are you kidding me? We just worked out!" The other girl naively replies with a huge smile, "Yea, but it only has fifteen calories!" Yes, fifteen calories of chemicals and additives (which spark a soft addiction for more chemicals, while mutating into immediate oxidation and inflammation). This is dangerous stuff. Calories are not the cornerstone measure of nutrition. Focus on Prana. Irrespective of calories, Prana comes from nutrient rich, bright, fresh, whole foods.

Not all Sugar is Created Equal. The sugar found in fruit is called fructose. This sugar is naturally balanced by the anti-oxidants, vitamins, and fibers that are also contained in the fruit. A teaspoon of white sugar can have the same amount of sweetness as a couple of grapes, but the body receives the information very differently. White sugar will create a fast acidic and inflammatory response in the body, while the sugar from the grapes will stay alkaline (acid free), and neutralized as a result of the collective chemistry. Pittas want to be especially cautious around acidic foods because they are already hot and acidic in nature. Get your sweetness from whole foods like root vegetables, fruits, dates, coconut water, whole grains, honey, jaggery, and even a dab of maple syrup.

> *"We all eat lies when our hearts are hungry."*
>
> **—Geneen Roth**

Fat Does Not Make You Fat. Good fats give us slow release, sustainable energy. Amino acids increase our cognitive functions, memory, and focus. Good fats provides us with brain fuel to feed Pitta. We need omega 3 and omega 6 fatty acids to support cognitive function and memory. Fats provide moisture to buffer the dryness of Vata in the joints, bones and intestines. Because fat is oily, it prevents crepitus (cracking joints) and constipation. There are thirty-six feet or so from the mouth to the anus. Fats work like internal WD-40, for our plumbing. Nothing gets stuck.

Fat is a building block of Kapha Dosha. Kapha provides cushion and insulation which protects our nervous systems and organs. As we know, we all have all three Doshas with in us, and all three Doshas are necessary to sustain life. Good fats come from sardines, salmon, nuts, seeds, avocados, coconut oil, olive oil, and ghee to name a few. We can customize how much fat we're consuming to harmonize with our unique mind-body make-up. For example, Vatas tolerate the most fat. Pitta's need less because of their already oily nature. And Kaphas require the least amount of fat.

Fat Free Will Not Make You Skinny. Fat free items are typically loaded with sugar and chemicals. Sugars process and store as fat, and chemicals boggle the metabolic hormones creating innumerable interferences between the brain and the gut. This type of miscommunication creates more cravings and Kapha-like imbalances such as weight gain, fluid retention, and excess phlegm. Chemicals create a disconnect between hunger and satiety. Sugar and chemicals provide no nutritional value. They do the opposite. They rob us of nourishment and satisfaction. I recently read a quote that stuck and continue to resonates, "When I see a sign that says, Fat Free, What I actually see is a sign that says Chemical Shit Storm." If something is not naturally fat free (like a pineapple or radish, for example), then you can guarantee chemicals and sugars have been added to replace the fat. You are better off eating the fat. Good fats have Prana, chemicals do not.

Processed and Artificial Food Do Not Process. We were designed to eat food. We have teeth to chew, taste buds to sense, saliva to swallow, and all the right equipment to break it down and use it effectively. We are programed to want, consume, digest, and eliminate food. The glitch occurs when we eat foods that are not in fact foods. Much of our food source has been contaminated with synthetic agents and additives. Our cultural atmosphere lends us to believe that something made it a factory, served from a box, and cooked in a microwave somehow qualifies as food. But this is not so. I love Michael Pollan's advice, "Don't eat anything incapable of rotting." If it will not rot, it will make us rot. Processed and artificial foods desecrate our micro-biome, which is the delicate, yet powerful ecosystem that dwells in our gut. The job of the micro-biome is to digest, absorb, and assimilate nutrients. Chemicals and additives make our micro-biome's job incredibly challenging to accomplish.

Eating processed and artificial foods leave the body in a state of perpetual confusion. Sugars and processed foods create exceedingly high amounts of immediate acidity and inflammation in the body. This leads to rapid oxidation. Oxidation happens when chemicals in food meet oxygen and metabolize in the body. This is a natural occurrence that can be reduced by eating fewer processed foods and mitigated by eating more antioxidants. Oxidative stress and free radical damage can make us feel rusty and wrinkly on the topical, and cellular level. Antioxidants help fight free radicals that are responsible for prematurely deteriorating the body. Typically the brighter the fruit or veggie—the more antioxidants it contains. Berries, cherries, artichokes, prunes, kidney beans, and the spice turmeric have the highest dosages of antioxidants. You will know something is high in antioxidants if maintains its brightness after being exposed to oxygen. For example, if you slice an apple and leave it on the counter for five minutes, the apple will turn brown. That is because only the skin on an apple is high in antioxidants. Conversely, if you slice a mango and leave it on the counter for five minutes, it will maintain it's vibrant hue. That is because the mango is loaded with antioxidants. Have you ever heard that squeezing lemon juice on food helps it keep it's color and reduces the brown tinge? My mom always uses this trick on party platters that will be out for a few hours. It works because lemon juice helps us by hindering oxidation. For this reason, it is good to drink hot water with lemon in the morning. It offers a nice flush of antioxidants.

Run from Anti-Nutrients. The term anti-nutrients is the fitting, and less than glamorous name attributed to food-like stuff that takes more than it gives. The very same products that were originally supposed to fuel us are actually draining us. Attractive packaging and concentrated flavors have caused our senses to override our logic. Allow me to illustrate with an analogy. Would you allow someone to come into your home and rob you of all the things that currently maintain your level of comfort and security? Of course not. What if that person was charming and gorgeous? What if they smothered you in tempting promises? Well, this is what our current market of "big food" does. They come into our lives with provocative, compelling, and tempting tales. Then they steal. Processed foods riddled with exaggeratedly strong synthetic flavors, chemicals, and additives rob us of nutrients and desecrate our gut flora (micro-biome).

There is a dangerous intersection where health and economics collide. Let us not be mistaken, food is a business and health care—more specifically, disease. Disease is an industry; a booming industry at that. To quote Dr.Timothy Ihrig from his Tedtalk, "We spend fifteen trillion dollars a year on the top 15% of our population who are most sick. The pharmaceutical industry is a 425 billion dollar industry, spending 1.6 billion dollars a year on marketing alone". I cannot help but think big food and big pharmacy are in cahoots. Medical schools are largely funded by pharmaceutical companies, yet medical students receive zero education on nutrition and the impact of food on health. Pharmaceutical and food companies have merged into massive conglomerates. I do not profess to know the motives behind the machines that drive this cumbersome issue. I personally have a hard time believing anyone enters the medical field without a tugging urge to help people. I do not think this the fault of our health care professionals. I recognize these people save lives. Medicine used in the right place at the right time is irreplaceable. But what I do know is, when it comes to my daily intake and wellness, I am not going to rely on big food companies to educate me on nutrition, nor I am not going to place all my confidence in the mainstream medical system to keep me healthy. Kale is cheap. Breath is free. Self-care is priceless, and our kitchens can become our front lines for prevention and healing.

Protect your Gut-Flora. The gut flora is a delicate and nuanced atmosphere of billions of bugs, bacteria, acids, and enzymes that help us digest, absorb, and assimilate nutrients. Did you know that one packet of Splenda (and like artificial sugars such as Equal and Sweet'n Low) will destroy 50% of your current gut flora, and frequent use of antibiotics will wipe out the good bugs that are trying to help you digest your food? We can support our gut flora with whole foods and spices. A tea made from equal parts ginger powder, cumin seeds, fennel seeds, and coriander seeds will help refurbish your gut flora. (Try Detox and Replenish Tea by Wellblends.) Taking a quality probiotic may be of additional value if your gut flora has been compromised.

New Times. New Measures. In the 1950's the average American spent 30% if their income on groceries and 10% on healthcare. Now days, the average American spends 10% of their income on groceries and 30% on healthcare. Why the flip? Hippocrates said, "Let food be thy medicine and thy medicine be thy food." There is a correlation between low quality food and low quality health, versus high quality food and higher qualities of health. In the 1950's no one thought to put on their Lululemon pants or tied up their Nike shoes for a Pilates class or a run. "Working out," as we think of it today was not on anyones' radar. People maintained their shape by performing daily duties like housework, farming, and yard maintenance. Now days, our jobs are primarily sedentary, and exercising has to built into our daily routines, or it just won't happen. Movement is no longer inherently woven into the designs of our days. In the 1950s people ate bacon for breakfast, apple pie for dessert and cooked with butter, yet their waistlines were slimmer. Where is the catch? Portions were smaller, and the ingredients—while not skimpy on calories and saturated fats, they were fresh. No chemicals. No diets. What is to take from all this?

We are Living in a New Paradigm. Never before in the history of human civilization has our food been sourced and distributed by aggregate industries. The amount of chemicals and additives that are funneled into our food sources are unprecedented. Our soil is denatured (stripped of minerals) and saturated in pesticides. This news is not to alarm you, it is probably not coming as a huge surprise. Taking a step back to see where we came from and where we at puts us at a vantage point to make smarter decisions that will improve our health. The health of our current food system and even the health of the planet request an overhaul. We are in a position of power. We can redirect our current trajectory. Every decision we make in regard to food will either endorse or protest the potentially calamitous trend. As we learned, we are a microcosm of the macrocosm, meaning our internal world is emulated in the external world. If we take better care of the world, we will take better care of ourselves. And if we take better care of ourselves, we will take better care of the planet. The relationship is synergistic, and we can start in our very own kitchens, favorite cafes, farmer's markets and grocery stores. Every seemingly little decision and act, performed by a number of people over an extended period of time will make a difference. For example, I recently resolved to only use canvas bags when grocery shopping. Plastic bags were taking over and polluting the space under my kitchen sink. I could not help but think about how they are polluting our oceans. Switching to canvas bags is one small, yet impactful way to exercise mindfulness and promote a positive shift.

> *"The wonderful thing about food is you get three votes a day. Every one of them has the potential to change the world."*
>
> **—Michael Pollan**

America is Overfed and Undernourished. What Are we Missing? Food consumes a large portion of our days. Whether we are eating, thinking about where we are going to eat, wishing we would not have eaten so much, going to the store to buy food, running to the deli for a sandwich, Starbucks for a coffee, grabbing a bite with a friend, lunch with an associate, enjoying or a candle light meal with our sweetie—food is undoubtedly on the menu. Thanks to mass media and a ravenous appetite for tips, trends, info, and quick fixes when it comes to our waistlines and health—this generation has been busting at the seams with information. But how reliable is the news we are being fed? Since food is an industry, the primary motivation of the industry is to make money.

The mainstream model places emphasis on providing profits for big business over nourishment for big America. As people become more aware of what is happening and more mindful in their choices—the dangerous trend of prioritizing profit over nourishment will capsize. One day, maybe the government will listen to the loud and responsible voices that are stating—if we feed our people properly, disease epidemics like cancer, heart disease and obesity will become less prevalent. Hello capitalism, making healthy food affordable is not just a moral obligation; it is fiscally sound.

> *"Good health makes a lot of sense, but it does not make a lot of dollars."*
>
> **—Dr. Andrew Saul**

The Mechanics: Understanding Food. There are plenty of faulty ideas around food. What to eat, how much to eat, and when to eat can seem ambiguous, but to make clear—food functions as a source of energy for the body, mind, and soul. The mechanics are simple. We should aim for balance between energy input and energy output. From a Western standpoint, we essentially need protein, carbohydrates, fats, vitamins, and minerals to support our physical and mental processes. Protein gives us brain and muscle power. Proteins do not need to be used immediately, they can be stored for future use. Healthy proteins include: legumes, seeds, nuts, fish and free-range/grass-fed/organic meat to name a few. You will also find protein in vegetables such as avocados, Brussels sprouts, broccoli, peas, spinach, and in lesser amounts potatoes, and corn.Carbohydrates give us readily available energy that we can quickly receive and burn. Carbohydrates come in the form of fruits, vegetables, and whole grains. Fats give us amino acids and brain power, lubrication and slow burn fuel. Fats give us a sense of satiety and staying power so we will not become immediately hungry after eating. Avoid refined carbohydrates like pasta and bread because they tend to be stripped of nutritional value, metabolized as sugar, and stored as sludgy fat. This is different from the good kind of fat, like the fat we get from avocados and quality oils. Sludgy fat that is born of sugar increases oxidation, congestion, and inflammation because it is not pure. For this reason, we should reduce white breads, refined, and processed grains. They are considered empty carbohydrates. These items are essentially bereft of Prana. Better options for whole grain include grains in their whole and complete form like, brown rice, basmati rice, millet, barley, jasmine rice, cuscus, or even sprouted bread like ezekiel bread—which can be found in the freezer section of your grocery store.

Eating a balanced meal that includes the cardinal components: proteins, fats, and carbohydrates will help harmonize the way food translates from your fork to satisfaction. A generous intake of these components will help set the stage for a Pranic rich meal. From this foundation of balance we can overlay Ayurvedic specifics.

> *"There is no such thing as junk food. There is junk. And there is food."*
>
> **—Dr. Mark Hyman**

The Healthy Cure is to Eat Whole Foods. Whole foods is not just a store. It is the name coined for foods that come directly from the earth. Whole foods include: grains, beans, nuts, seeds, fruits, veggies, organic/free range/grass fed meats, ghee and honey. Whole foods are dense in the nutrients, vitamins, and minerals that replenish our cells, organs, and tissues. You know a whole food when you see it because the food looks remarkably similar to how you would see it in a nature. For example, a snack consisting of a banana and a handful of almonds would be considered a whole foods snack whereas a fat free "banana-almond" snack bar is not. To boost our health on a cellular level, we want the gap between where our food came from and the way it appears on our plate to be relatively slender.

Be Cautious of Labels. Labels can be deceiving. If you have been fooled by fancy marketing, do not feel bad. I have been duped too. Marketing is savvy. A box of cereal that claims to be full of fiber and calcium, while being low in calories and fat free should not excite you. This cereal is likely loaded with sugar and additives. Any nutritional content was stripped away in the processing and then "fortified" (added back in) in the factory. Be wary of labels that make bold claims. In fact, the best foods do not even need a label. Fruits and vegetables are often naked, completely label free.

Shopping Tips. Try to shop at a Farmer's Market or Organic Co Op if possible. In grocery stores, stay on the perimeter because most of the canned, bagged, and boxed food that have been heavily processed are located in the center. Allow fruits and veggies to consume the biggest proportion of your shopping cart and your receipt.

Cooking Methods. Microwaves nuke food. Nuke, like a bomb, as in destroy. See where I am going with this? Microwaves zap nutritional content out of the food. Frozen meals and microwaved foods are a part of the reason America is overfed and undernourished (frozen foods are particularly disruptive for Vata types because as the frozen molecules melt, they create gas and bloating). We can eat a meal, but if the meal is nutritionally empty due to the preparation method, we will crave more because frankly—our bodies did not receive what they needed. You can use a microwave to heat food if that is your best available option. But, avoid using the microwave to cook food. As an experiment, I cooked one sweet potato in the oven and one in the microwave. The sweet potato that came out of the over was soft, bright, and tasted incredibly sweet. The other, from the microwave was dry, pale, and bland to taste. The microwave is the last resort. If needed; use the microwave only to heat your food; not to cook your food. Never microwave from a plastic container. The plastic leech into your food. Use a glass or ceramic container instead.

> *"People are fed by the food industry, which pays no attention to health...and there are treated by the health industry, which pays no attention to food."*
>
> **—Wendell Berry**

Avoid frying food. Fried food contributes to heart disease, obesity, diabetes, and just a flat out yucky feeling. This is especially true for Kapha Dosha, who tend to have a slower metabolism and harder time processing fatty foods. Try to grill, bake, sauté, or roast food. Ghee and coconut oil are best for cooking because they have a high smoke point, meaning they can get very hot with minimal change to their molecular structure. Heat alters the chemistry thereby making something that was healthy carcinogenic, or toxic. This happens with olive oil. Olive oil is very good for you, but should be used for cooking at low heat or drizzled on before serving.

The Breakdown on Confusing Terms

- Organic—This mean it was grown without pesticides. These foods are without debate healthier.
- All Natural—This is a fad term that has no relevance. It is used to generate sales.
- Gluten Free—This means there is no gluten. Gluten is a specific protein often found in grains, specifically wheat. Gluten in of itself was not originally harmful. We have been eaten gluten for centuries. One theory surrounding the epidemic of recent digestive issues in reference to gluten is that years ago we had a lot more variety in our food source. Our digestive system was designed to breakdown a variety of grains, but nowadays agriculture is produced on such a large scale that genetically modified crops have overtaken fields, and we have lost the diversification that our digestive system demands. The inability to digest gluten can exasperate celiac disease, autoimmune disease, and neurological imbalances. Many of our grains are now milled into a white flour that is essentially nutrient free, so it is best to avoid it when possible. (Pitta types can usually digest gluten because they have strong digestive fires. Gluten may create gas and bloating for Vatas and mucus and weight gain for Kapha types).

» GMO-genetically modified organism. This method is used in pharmaceutical drugs, medicines, and agriculture. Wheat, soy and corn are typically GMO. There is much controversy around the impact of eating GMO foods. We are part of the first generation of people consuming mostly GMO foods. Without consent, we have become part of a global experiment. The definitive results are to be determined. To play is safe—avoid GMO foods.

"Food is not just a calorie, it is information. It talks to your DNA and tells it what to do. The most powerful tool to change your health, environment and entire world is on your fork."

—Dr. Mark Hyman

PAUSE FOR AFFIRMATION

"I am compassionately aware of how food influences me. I choose to energize and nourish my body and mind with wholesome foods."

"The key to creating health is figuring out the cause of the problem and then finding the right conditions for the body and soul to thrive."

—Mark Hyman

As the saying goes, "You are what you eat." But I'd say, "You are what you think, and what you think drives what you eat...so you are what you think." Too Dr.Suess? Here's my point—if food issues were actually about food no one would have an issue to begin with. Why? Because food isn't complicated. Food in of itself isn't good or bad. It's not emotional. Food in of itself is not a reward or punishment. Food is not a philosophy or religion. Food is in its most natural state, nourishment, energy, and sustenance. Food is an appendage of Mother Earth. And Mother Earth did not create sugar addictions, an overwhelming data dump of trends/diets/fads, and Mother Earth most certainly did not create pains associated with body image. "Healthcare" (I put that in quotes because I don't believe all health paradigms have our best interest in mind), beauty, and marketing industries generated and perpetuated our dilemmas with food. Social conditioning and culture exasperated our woes. Einstein said, "No problem can be solved at the same level of consciousness that created it." Our conundrums with food are actually toxic extensions of industry and marketing. The solution to our food problems and the passage towards cultivating a healthy relationship with food will not be found through industry nor marketing. The solution will come from Mother Earth.

CHAPTER ELEVEN

Ayurvedic Nutrition

"While forbidden fruit is said to taste sweeter, it usually spoils faster."

—Abigail Van Buren

QUALITIES. AYURVEDA DOES not speak in terms of calories, carbs, proteins, and fats. Nutrition is defined in terms of its qualities, tastes, and digestive effect. Just as qualities are present within the Doshas, qualities are present within foods. Understanding the qualities of food will assist in helping us choose foods that will balance the qualities of our constitution. The qualities of light, dry, rough, quick and subtle are catabolic, meaning reducing. They lighten us. These qualities balance Kapha Dosha. The qualities heavy, moist, smooth, slow, oily, and stable are anabolic, meaning building. They ground us. These qualities are best for Pitta and Vata. If you look at a salad with fresh lettuce, shaved carrots, sliced bell peppers and tomatoes, drizzled with balsamic vinegar you will see the qualities present in the salad are light, dry, rough, quick and subtle. These qualities will increase Vata.

If you look at a bowl of sweet potato chili you will note the qualities are heavy, moist, slow, smooth, oily, and stable. These qualities will increase Kapha. In short, when you sit down and look at your plate of food. Recognize the qualities. If you have a Vata imbalance; say you have not been sleeping well, you feel anxious, and you have been constipated, you do not want to look at your plate and see a salad with carrots, hummus and crackers. These light, dry and quick qualities will only feed the imbalance. You would be better off with a plate of sautéed zucchini and a cup of brown rice drizzled with olive oil for instance.

We apply the principle of opposites to create balance. Character Sketch: Meet Alice… If Alice has a Vata imbalance. Her skin and hair are dry. Her colon is dry and rough—leading to constipation. Her sleep is light—creating insomnia. Her bones are light and dry—responsible for crepitus. And her mind is subtle and quick—creating anxiety. With a Vata imbalance, Alice wants to avoid foods that share the qualities that are currently contributing to her imbalance. So, Alice will avoid dry/rough/quick/subtle and light foods. Instead she will have moist/smooth/slow/stable and heavy foods. What this looks like for Alice:

» Alice will swap her raw salad for sautéed veggies. Vata types should sauté using plenty of ghee or coconut oil and cooking spices like ginger, turmeric, and black pepper to support digestion. (Try Agni, by Wellblends)

» She will replace her crackers with brown rice.

» And she will substitute her usual snack of popcorn for an avocado instead.

The foods Alice shifted to are all moist, smooth, slow, stable, and heavy. These foods will bring Alice into balance. This exemplifies how we use the kitchen as medicine.

Character Sketch: Meet Sam... If Sam has a Pitta imbalance. Her skin is oily, creating acne. Her mind is sharp, breeding frustration and irritability. Her body is light, propelling her tendency to run around trying to get too many things done at once, and her stools are loose—due to too much moisture. Sam will avoid foods that are oily/sharp/light and moist. Instead, she will have foods that are cooling/dry and heavy.

What this looks like for Sam:

- » Sam will swap her chicken wings with buffalo sauce for baked chicken.
- » She will exchange her spicy tomato soup for a more drying lentil soup and quinoa.
- » And she will substitute her usual snack of bell peppers in jalapeño hummus for dried fruits.

Now the foods that Sam is eating are cooler, dryer, and heavier. This will bring Sam back into balance.

Character Sketch: Meet Marta... Marta has a Kapha imbalance. Her head is cloudy due to a heavy, stable quality. Her energy is low due to a slow and dull qualities, and her allergies are acting up because of moist and sticky qualities that are present. Marta will avoid foods that are heavy/stable/dull/slow/sticky and moist. Instead she will have foods that favor warm/light/quick/subtle and drying qualities. What this looks like for Marta:

- » Marta will replace my macaroni and cheese with asparagus, cooked with ghee and a cup of millet.
- » She will swap steak for fish.
- » And she will substitute her usual snack of frozen yogurt for an apple and herbal tea.

Marta is now enjoying lighter, quicker, and warmer qualities. These food choices will help bring Marta back into balance.

To be fair, when I first met Ayurveda I was not ready to change my food. The way I had been eating felt easy and safe. It gave me a sense of control. Augmenting my beliefs and behaviors around food took time to adopt and adapt. When I initially learned about Ayurvedic nutrition, I ate mostly cold cereals, fat free milk, lettuce, fat free salad dressings and granola bars. Once I learned that the qualities of these foods I was consuming were Vata aggravating I softened to the idea of implementing slow steady changes. I swapped my cold cereals and fat free milk for oatmeal made with almond milk. I traded in my lettuce and fat free (chemical) dressings for sautéed veggies, and I exchanged my granola bars for dates. The changes did not require monumental leaps in content or time, but the effects were drastic. My Vata imbalances (constipation, scanty or absent periods, interrupted sleep, and anxiety) were relieved simply by eating more warm and grounding foods. Foods that contained the exact opposite qualities of my imbalanced state.

> *"Somedays you eat salad and go to the gym, somedays you eat cupcakes and refuse to put on pants. It is called balance."*
>
> **—Unknown**

Tastes. There are six tastes. You may have experienced that when you eat a savory meal, you want something sweet to top it off. Or after a sweet indulgence, you want something salty or spicy. These patterns are generated by the bodies desire to achieve balance. By eating all six tastes in every meal you will feel satisfied and curb cravings. Initially, recognizing taste can prove more challenging than one might think. Packaged foods are packed with high concentrations of artificial flavors that have a way of stripping and desensitizing the taste buds. Our taste buds regenerate every ten days, so be patient as you become re-sensitized to natural flavors. If whole foods seem bland, then your taste buds have become accustomed to fabricated tastes, they are numb to natural tastes. After eating whole foods for a week or two, you will come to appreciate the burst of flavors contained in natural foods.

The standard American diet (with the acronym, SAD... Is that a coincidence?) The typical American diet is largely dependent on the tastes sweet, sour, and salty. Cuisine in the West runs pretty skimpy on the tastes pungent, bitter, and astringent. Part of the reason why Americans might be so in love with coffee is that it satisfies the need for bitter—that we are otherwise neglecting. Imbalances in our eating habits tastes in every meal to feel satisfied. Mental and physical disparities can be attributed to missing this key principle: We need all six tastes to achieve balance.

Each Taste is Responsible for a Primary Action

Sweet: Builds tissues and calm the nerves. Vatas tend to be thin and nervous, so sweet is great for Vata Dosha. Sweet counter balances the light and hot nature of Pitta, so sweet is also good for Pitta Dosha.

Sour: Cleanses channels and increases absorption of minerals. Sour is a building taste, so it is good for Vata Dosha.

Salty: Improves taste of food, lubricates tissues and stimulates digestion. The lubrication effect of salt counterbalances the dry nature of Vata, so salty tastes are good for Vata Dosha.

Pungent: Stimulates digestion and metabolism. Kapha Dosha needs to be stimulated, so pungent, or spicy taste is good for Kapha types.

Bitter: Detoxifies and lightens tissues. Kapha Dosha will benefit from the lightening effect of bitter foods. Bitter is also very cooling, so Pitta types should also try bitter foods.

Astringent: Absorbs water, tightens tissues and dries fat. Kapha types tend to have excess moisture and fat, so they should enjoy astringent foods. Pitta Dosha is also moist and will gravitate toward astringent tastes to find balance.

Best Tastes Per Dosha. As we learned, we should all consume all six tastes to feel balanced and satiated, but we should maximize particular tastes according to our Dosha. Remember, you should eat in accordance to your body type and current state. For example, I may have a Vata mind and a Kapha body. In that case, I will eat for my Kapha body type. Or, my True Nature may be Pitta Dosha but right now I have a Vata imbalance in my body (for example, I recently lost weight and suffer from constipation). In this case, I will eat for my Vata body-type imbalance.

To Review:

- » Vata Dosha should gravitate toward primarily sweet, sour and salty tastes.
- » Pitta Dosha should lean towards sweet, bitter and astringent tastes.
- » Kapha Dosha should eat mostly pungent, bitter and astringent tastes.

What this looks like on your plate: Vatas may enjoy more grains, root vegetables (like squash and sweet potato), sweet fruits (like melons and mangoes), sour fruits (citrus fruits like oranges and grapefruit), seafood, nuts and seeds. Pittas may enjoy more bitter vegetables like leafy greens, and cruciferous vegetables (like broccoli and cauliflower), beans, grains, sweet fruits (like watermelon and coconut), astringent fruits (like berries, apples and pomegranates) and herbal teas. Kaphas may enjoy more leafy greens (kale, arugula, mustard and dandelion greens), calciferous vegetables (like broccoli and cauliflower), astringent fruits (like cranberries and pomegranates), spicy foods (like onions, black pepper, chilis and wasabi) and will benefit from the bitter taste of coffee and astringent taste of black tea. If Kapha types should want to eat grains that should enjoy buckwheat, millet and barley because these grains are slightly more astringent than sweet (they have a more heating and drying effect on the body). Now you can see why we needed to address our modern stand point and the necessity of removing processed foods prior to enhancing our awareness with these empowering principles. Could you imagine if I would have suggested to someone who eats a standard American diet of fast food and microwave meals… "Hey there! You have a

Vata imbalance so you should eat sweet, sour and salty foods". That person might have be like, "Bingo!", Quickly run to the vending machine for a sweet snickers bars, a bag of sour patch kids and a bag of salty chips and think, "Nailed it!" Not quite. While technically, that satisfies the request for sweet, sour, and salty, the extreme and artificial nature of the tastes would have accentuated the imbalance.

The body is of a natural, intelligent design. It has a specific language and responds to food that speaks the same natural and intelligent language. Try this analogy on for size. You speak English, but feeding the body processed food is like someone trying to speak to your body in in Czech. If you do not speak Czech. It will not matter how slow or fast, much or little, loud or softly the person speaks you will still be wildly confused and unable to comprehend because it is all together unfamiliar. The body recognizes processed foods as foreign—totally alien. Eating whole foods, real food, food from the earth guarantees that your body and your food are speaking the same language. Be patient, learning a new language does not happen without time and will.

Post Digestive Effect. Foods create temperature shifts in the body. We are not talking directly talking about the temperature of the food, but rather its post digestive effect. For example, a chili pepper cold be cold to the touch, whereas when you put it in the body it feels very hot. Conversely, herbal tea made with mint and cilantro could feel hot on the tongue, but creates a cooling effect in the body.

Heating & Cooling. Vata and Kapha Dosha are both cool Doshas, so they respond well to heating foods and spices like garlic, ginger, and black pepper, whereas Pitta Dosha is hot, and reacts well with cooling foods like melon, mint, and aloe. Everyone does well with cooked foods rather than raw. This is because it is easier to break down cooked food because the enzyme releasing activity has already been initiated. In fact, the brain capacity of human beings increased once man discovered the ability to make fire and cook his or her food. It takes a lot of energy to cook and break down food in the gut. If we externally cook the food, we save internal energy, so the energy can be used elsewhere—like the mind. It is advisable not to overcook food because it is possible to cook at the nutrients out. Food should maintain a similar color and texture to its raw version, even when it is cooked. This way you know the food is still loaded with essential nutrients. If you really want raw food—drink ginger tea with black pepper to rev up your digestive fire prior to eating the raw food. That way when the food reaches the gut your digestive powers will be prepped at full throttle. Applying the principle, "Opposites Create Balance" teaches us that it is best to eat cool foods in hot weather. If it is cold outside and you are eating cold food, you will experience an imbalance.

A Word on Juicing and Smoothies… There is nothing wrong with enjoying pure, fresh juices or smoothies. Just be mindful of your most predominant Dosha and the season of the year to determine just how often you should be juicing or partaking in smoothies. No Doshic type should consume a lot of cool liquids in the fall or early winter because the air is cold, light and dry, so you need warm, heavy and moist foods to maintain balance. Generally speaking, Vatas should consume more warm and grounding meals over juices and smoothies year round. Pittas do well with juices and smoothies, but will need a bit more substance to fill them up due to their quick and powerful metabolisms. Pittas can add ground flaxseed and chia seeds to their smoothies to add staying power. Kapha types will benefit the most from juicing, and drinking light smoothies because liquid meals are quick and easy to digest. All three Doshas should add ginger, turmeric, and like heating spices to their smoothies and juices to aid in digestion, reduce inflammation, and gain a generous dose of antioxidants. You could easily add ½-1 tsp of Golden Milk powder to your smoothies and juices for both taste and vitality. Juices and smoothies are convenient to eat on the go. With that said, do not be tempted to abandon the mindful eating component that marries healthy food to a healthy body.

Agni, the Digestive Fire. We are what we eat, but more importantly—we are what we digest. Our ability to digest our food gives thanks to our Agni, or digestive fire. This is the quality of our gastric juices such as, hydrochloric acid, bile, and digestive enzymes. The strength of your fire determines how well you break down food, assimilate nutrients, and eliminate waste. Lets say three people sit down to eat the same exact meal, at the same exact time, in the same exact proportions. Person A has a strong digestive fire and is able to metabolize the food without any issues. Person B has a sharp digestive fire, meaning their GI is acidic with a presence of overpowering bile. This person may experience acid indigestion or heartburn. While Person C has a weak digestive fire. For person C, the same meal may make them feel uncomfortably full, it can create gas or sit with them, feeling like a brick in the gut for hours upon hours. Same food, Same time, Same place. Different experience. This is all due to the Agni, or digestive fire.

Our goal is to have a strong and balanced fire.

Signs you have a strong and balance digestive fire: (Ayurveda refers to this as, Sama Agni)

» You get hungry.

» You have a good appetite.

» You are able to digest your food without gas/ bloating, or heaviness.

» You are able to eliminate daily.

Signs you have a weak digestive fire: (Ayurveda refers to this as, Manda Agni)

» You do not get hungry.

» You have a weak appetite.

» You experience gas/bloating, or heaviness after eating.

» You do not eliminate daily.

Indications that your digestive fire may be too strong, or you're eating aggravating (hot, acidic, sharp) foods: (Ayurveda refers to this as Tikshna Agni)

» You are ravenous.

» You are hungry shortly after eating.

» You experience acid reflux, heartburn, or GERD.

» You have loose stools multiple times a day.

Remember to meet yourself where you are. We can only begin from our own personal starting point. I find this analogy to be helpful. Say you are going to clean a room, and this particular room happens to be in complete disarray. They floor is crowded with clothes and belongings. There is soot on the windows, cobwebs on the fan, and clutter everywhere. You would not narrow in on one little trinket and start dusting the trinket. First you would tackle the big stuff. You would organize the clutter, and resolve the more pressing obstacles first. Changing your diet is similar. Begin by focusing on the most area that request your direct attention. Start by eating more whole foods. Approaching the more subtle nuances will be easier once the core topic has been remedied. The hands down, absolute, most important aspect is to be kind to yourself.

Meal prepping makes life easier…Let's face it, we're all busy. In a perfect world we could eat wholesome, freshly prepared meals three times a day every day. Realistically, that's unlikely. Meal prepping allows us to anticipate our needs and meet them by being proactively prepared. I recommend meal prepping once a week, twice if possible. Here are a few staple meal prep suggestion per Dosha. These are items you could make on Sunday and eat from all week. Or ideally, make half of the food for the week on Sunday, and do a second round of meal prepping on Wednesday or Thursday. That way everything stays even more fresh. Once your main items are prepared you can create bowls and a variety of dishes from the same set of components.

Vata: a pot of brown rice, a few roasted chicken breasts, a few filets of baked salmon, a crock pot of squash soup and half a dozen sweet potatoes. Also have on hand avocados, dates, figs, fresh greens (for sautéing), and overnight oats (for breakfast).

You can play with variations. Make a bowl of sautéed green, brown rice, and chicken one day. Have a sweet potato and piece of salmon the next. Have a bowl of soup, a cup of oats with dates and figs, or brown rice with salmon—garnished with thin slices of avocado. You see, once everything is at your fingertip it's easy to construct wholesome meals without overthinking or overworking. You'll feel grounded and nourished by these foods.

Pitta: a crockpot of lentil soup, a pot of basmati rice, a few filets of baked fresh water fish, spaghetti squash, and a big wok of stir-fried greens. Also have on hand: carrots and hummus to snack on, apples, watermelon, and coconut milk to add to the stir-fry to make curry. You could have lentils over basmati one day, a bowl with veggies, rice and fish the next day, a plate of spaghetti squash with olive oil the next, a stir-fry coconut curry with rice, and nice fruit bowl for breakfast or as a snack. Once your sticked up, it's easy to feel refreshed and satiated by your options.

Kapha: a pot of black beans, a pot of quinoa, sautéed bell peppers and onions, a few roasted chicken breasts, a tray of roasted Brussel sprouts, and a crock pot of vegetable soup. Also have, berries, fresh greens, and hot sauce on hand. You can make a bowl with black beans and sautéed veggies (add hot sauce to your liking) one day, a plate of roasted chicken with Brussel sprouts the next, a bowl of veggie soup the following, and a smoothie with berries and fresh greens for breakfast as well. Once you have plenty of light, warming foods prepared you can play with pairings and find what makes you feel best.

"Do the best you can until you know better. Then when you know better, do better."

—Maya Angelou

PAUSE FOR AFFIRMATION

"I am listening to what my body needs. I am choosing foods that balance and satisfy the loving request of my body."

CHAPTER TWELVE

Feed Your Spirit and Your Belly

"Tell me what you eat and I will tell you who you are."

—Jean Anthelme Brillat-Savarin

APPETITE AND SATIETY. We understand our appetites are directly related to the strength of our personal Agni. Ideally you want a solid appetite. There are several barometers that serve to inform you if your digestive system is functioning well or not.

1. You get hungry.
2. You feel satisfied after you eat.
3. You feel light and have increased physical and mental energy after eating.
4. Several hours later, you are hungry again.
5. You have a bowel movement at least once a day.

The first measure of good digestion is the ability to feel hunger. We often deny our hunger, either through restrictions or distractions. It is wise to respect the feedback the body constantly provides. Feeling satisfied is the second measure of good digestion. Eating balanced meals create satiety. This should include:

1. Sources of protein, carbs (vegetables quality as carbohydrates) and fat. For example: a piece of fish and a roasted sweet potato drizzled in olive oil. The fish is protein, the sweet potato is a carbohydrate and the olive oil is fat. Perfect.
2. All six tastes.
3. The correct portion in relation to your Agni. If you are hungry, eat more. If you are not hungry, eat less. I know it sounds so obvious when we see it on paper, however, it is commonly overlooked principle. The mind and desires can override the very clear and intelligent signals of the body. Listen to your body.

"The inability to love and accept yourself and your humanity is at the heart of many illnesses. To be loved and accepted, you must start by loving yourself. If you have traits that you consider unlovable, you must love them anyway…it is a paradox."

—Christine Northrup

Emotional Eating. I could just skirt around this subject, or sweep it under the rug, but not addressing a problem will not make it less of a problem. Looking at the conundrum as a lifestyle classroom to learn, can invert a curse into a blessing. In Chinese the word 'crisis' is composed of the two Chinese characters, respectively denoting 'danger' and 'opportunity'. Shedding light on what feels like a personal crisis can grant us the power to turn a potential danger into a real opportunity to experience healing and a palpable change in our lives. I want to address emotional eating because according to Ayurveda, diseases are often caused by repressed emotions. This is a delicate subject. Emotional eating can create turmoil and heartache for those of us who have been there. I am not going to claim that myself, Ayurvedic tools, or any single tool for that matter can correct this issue on its own. Our relationship with food is so immediate and intimate. Outside influences can give us perspective, but true healing comes from self-knowledge and self-love. It is remarkably personal journey. Goodness, if it were easy to correct, so many of us would not have to wrestle with it. To quote Wayne Dyer, "Nothing good comes from just feeling bad." It is our responsibility and within our power to gather truths and find a team to support us when an issue like emotional eating comes to clouds our lives. I love this idea of gathering a team while we are well. It is common practice to wait until we are sick to form a support group, but by then our support group may be an oncologist, physical therapist, or the hospital nurses. Why not create a fellowship around wellness and health while we are healthy?

Nutrition comes from the word nourish. It is easy to reach for food in effort to fill an unmet void or need. But according Ayurveda food should not be misused as a control mechanism through deprivation or over indulgence. Food is meant to keep us alive, our bodies energetic, and our minds sharp. To have reverence and respect for the food that nourishes you is one way to have reverence and respect for yourself. The Chinese say, "Disease enters through the mouth". We should take care to provide ourselves with proper nourishment to satisfy our bellies, support our daily activities, and replenish to achieve appropriate levels of energy. Any more or any less will not serve as medicine, but as a hindering vice. If we find ourselves routinely reaching for food or avoiding food in efforts to satiate an unmet need that is a clue to take pause and have a deeper look at what we really want. I often remind myself to nourish myself verses feed myself. There is a distinct difference. Feeding myself could be shoveling in calories so I don't pass out. Nourishing myself requires more personal inquiry and conscious actions.

Stress Eating… Who among us has not reached for food in effort to alleviate stress? This is a common habit. A long day, ornery kids, a massive project, impending deadlines, a fight with a friend, a subtle insult, you name it. Food seems to always be this safe haven; a retreat from the baggage, opinions, request, demands, or expectations of others. But food is not a magic bullet that will swallow daily woes. The Buddhist revere food as daily sustenance. A source of fuel to sustain life. Not too little, not too much. Food as sustenance is correct. Food is not meant to be an intoxicant, sedative or distraction from the colors of life.

In times of stress a primitive process takes place. Under stress our body goes into fight or flight mode. Evolutionarily, the body recognizes stress as the presence of a threat such as a tiger. The body is prepared to run from the tiger, or whatever it is that is creating the stress. At this point systems such as the libido, or in this case the digestive system shut down. We clearly do not need to have sex, or a snack if we biologically think it is time to run from a tiger. In such, under stress all of our blood flow is diverted away from the digestive tract, and redirected to escape the threat. Essentially, our ability to digest food is postponed in times of stress. This is not a good time to eat. Food can give us a sense of comfort because we are consuming something that is familiar. We know it is safe. But, we can get this same sense of comfort from "re-consuming" anything that is familiar. We can watch a movie we have seen several times, visit a park we frequently visit, listen to our favorite song, visit our familiar meditation oasis, or even smell familiar scents. Next time you are tempted to absolve stress with food, try to consume an alternate form of familiarity and comfort—such as, your favorite movie, song, meditation or sanctuary. Stress eating can be tempered by distracting yourself with one of the healthy examples above, or you can simply drink a cup of hot water and take three deep breaths. From there, if you do choose to eat, it will be from a place of conscious choice, rather than unconscious reflex. If you have meal prepped, and stocked your environment with healthful options you will be more likely to eat Pranic—rich, nutrient-rich foods that will provide relief verses destruction. Make no mistake about it, eating a sleeve of Oreos or bag of skittles will not make stress dissolve. It will however, make our ability to consciously respond to stress very challenging. The gunk in "treats" pollutes our mind-body, resulting in brain fog, fatigue, and discomfort. We are now aware of better options, and we deserve to partake in the options that do not prologue disease, but rather truly restore ease. Real food brings ease. Junk food does not. However, remember that love is the most medicinal ingredient in our lives. It is better to eat junk food with love in your heart, than eat wholesome food with vengeful thoughts in your mind. I'll never forget my Ayurveda Nutrition teacher said, "I would rather you eat McDonalds under an oak tree; feeling grateful for your food and your life, than eat a wholesome meal while fighting with your family and watching the news." Ayurveda understands that what we're thinking and feeling impact the alchemy of digestion and nourishment. Yes, the content of our food is being consumed. But so is the content in our minds. Be loving...especially towards yourself.

> *"Go and love someone exactly as they are. And then watch how quickly then transform into the greatest, truest version of themselves. When one feels seen and appreciated in their own essence, one is instantly empowered."*
>
> **—Wes Angelozzi**

Self-Shame to Self-Love. I met with a client and friend who had suffered from an eating disorder, and was wildly familiar with patterns of emotional eating. Our conversations always stemmed from vulnerability and truth. We discussed ideas like shame and guilt. I recall one particular session where we realized emotional eating could be transformed from an act of self-shame into an act of self-love. I suggested that when she felt these episodes of intense emotion, the urge to binge, ensued by the inevitable wake of guilt and shame brewing—that she first pause. Being the wise and intuitive women she is, she could sense these feeling bubbling up. She committed to transforming adverse moments into moments of love and nourishment. From there on out, the moment she thought she was going to binge, she got out a plate, cloth napkin, and her finest utensils. She selected her donut, cookies, cake, or other pleasure of choice, and mindfully served a modest potion onto her plate or into her bowl. She sat down, lit a candle, and shut her eyes. She took a few deep breaths and reminded herself how loved and worthy she is. She opened her eyes, took a big bite—followed by many more slow, conscious, loving bites. When the plate was empty or the bowl was clean she put her fork down and said, "I deserved that. I love myself."

This sweet woman was able to not only overcome a tumultuous struggle. She was able to use the power of love and care to turn something dark into something strikingly light. There is an indescribable component to healing that cannot be read, learned, or even prescribed. There is an intuitive voice, a connection, a truth that when given the space and time comes through, and that light guides the way.

"The sooner we heal it within ourselves, the sooner we will also free our daughters."

—Christine Northrup

Body Image. So much of what we know about food is generated and perpetuated around achieving a certain body image, versus achieving a certain standard of health. Fat free pretzels with diet coke, a couple cigarettes, and a cup of coffee might get you skinny, but they will not make you healthy. We should focus on health, because healthy is the best kind of beautiful. We do not need to fit into a specific size pair of jeans. Who cares if you never fit into the "skinny jeans" that have been sitting in the back of your closet for the last five years? Wearing those jeans probably will not make you feel more accomplished, valued or loved for more than a nostalgic five minutes. But becoming comfortable in your skin feeling grateful for the way your muscles hug your bones, your lips curl up to smile, and you toes spread to find balance will give you the confidence to love and accomplish whatever it is you want.

"The function of the body is to carry the brain around."

—Thomas Edison

The body is smart. Human beings were designed to be aesthetically pleasing. Look at a baby. They are irresistibly cute. It does not matter how much they cry or dirty their diapers, we love them anyway because their cuteness is enchanting. Adults have the same appeal. It is only the misperception, fear, and insecurity that would have us believe it any other way. As you get in the groove of making choices that align with your True Nature, your True Nature will shine forth and you will see—you are absolutely beautiful. Dr. Vasant Lad says, "Behind every emotion is love." Please, love your body.

> *"Good nutrition and vitamins do not directly cure disease, the body does. You provide the raw materials and the inborn of your body makes the repairs."*
>
> **—Andrew W. Saul**

Food Can Illustrate the Way you Want to Feel. When you look at your plate with the mindset, "You are what you eat", make sure your food illustrates the way you want to feel. If your food looks bland, you will likely feel bland. If your food looks heavy, you may feel heavy. If your food looks vibrant, fresh and balanced—you will likely feel vibrant, fresh and balanced. Allow food to embody the qualities you wish to embody. I aim for my food to look balanced, creative, and satisfying. Choose the words that describe what you desire for yourself then think of your plate as a canvas for which you can draw a self portrait.

Cravings. By eating a balanced meal with all six tastes you will evade cravings. Avoid chemicals, sugars, and processed food that send your blood sugar through disorienting peaks and valleys. Skipping meals and overindulging will only accentuate patterns of cravings. If your Doshas are in balance and you have a craving, it could be a craving you can trust. This could be an actual and relevant feedback from the body. Women often crave chocolate around their menstrual cycle because chocolate is full of magnesium and zinc, two essential minerals the body requires to replenish blood. If you are craving red meat you may need iron. However, most cravings are psychological. If a craving should arise, you and you choose to indulge, partake in whatever it is you are craving with gratitude, free from guilt. Our thoughts about ourselves and what we are eating influence the way we physiologically and physiological digest food. Eating a cookie while feeling guilty will not satisfy your craving and support your wellbeing. Whereas eating the cookie with gratitude and respect towards yourself and circumstance can certainly support your wellbeing. Cravings are the mind-body way of indicating that a need is unmet. The genius of the human body knows just what it needs to function. In many cases it can even produce what it needs on its own. For example, it produces bile and enzymes to help us break down food, synovial fluid to keep our joints lubricated, white blood cells to keep our immune system strong, hormones to keep our moods balanced, anti-inflammatories to keep us ache free and so on. The mind-body communicates through neuropeptides and cellular communication.The mind-body relationship as an interconnected system. For example, you see a commercial for a warm blueberry muffin and all of a sudden your have a sudden hunger for a blueberry muffin. You walk past a cafe and smell coffee and in an instant you have a strong urge to grab a coffee. You have a thought that makes you miss your mom and now you are craving creamy macaroni and cheese, like the one she used to make. So many of the things our body wants are initiated in the mind, and so many things the mind desires are signaled from a bodily cue. Learning to watch your thoughts and listen to your body is the first step in learning to understand and manage cravings.

"Eating is a natural way to feel happy. Overeating isn't."

—Deepak Chopra

Balance and Portions. The Okinawans have one of the longest life expectancies on the planet. The people of this Japanese city live upwards of 100 years. When asked what their secret is, they reported, "We eat until we're 80% full. " Never more, rarely less. Just 80% capacity. I thought this was very clever, but when I went to put it into action, I realized I had no idea what 80% was, or 50%, or 30%, or any other percent for that matter felt like. My gauge for how much I was eating in relation to my digestive space was undetectable. Learning to measure your digestive strength, capacity, limits, and ideal sensations of satisfaction requires time, practice and considerable awareness.

Ayurveda suggests to eat until your stomach is 1/3 full of food, 1/3 full of liquids and 1/3 left empty. We need the empty space to allow the gastric juices to move around, massage, and breakdown the matter. If the GI is crammed tight with matter it will take an extended amount of time to breakdown and will likely create indigestion. As a model to establish a sensible portion size, take your two hands in prayer—open your palms with the pinky side of the hand still touching. That's your perfect portion. The size of your hands is relative to the size of your individual body, so the amount of food will vary from person to person. You should take your digestive strength (Agni) into consideration as well. A stronger Agni, can digest more food.

Keep in mind that not all portion increments are created equal. For example, one cup of lasagna is not the same as one cup of sautéed kale. For dense foods, like red meat, cheese, heavy grains, items with cream sauce and hearty root vegetables keep the portion sizes under one fist full. (Ideally, animal products should be kept to a bare minimum, and Kapha types should avoid these foods all together). If you are eating very light foods, like sautéed vegetables or salads, you could easily consume larger quantities without taxing your digestive system. Heavy foods that contain more protein and fat have staying power. They will keep you full longer so you do not need as much. Whereas light carbohydrates, like fruits and vegetables provide easy access, short term fuel, meaning you will need more to stay full longer.

Mindful Eating. Ayurveda suggests that we are not only what we eat, but also when, how and why. We all live busy modern lives. We may not have the resources to completely perfect the content of everything we put into our mouths. We may not have the time and flexibility to eat our meals at the exact right time each day, but what we do have is the awareness to eat mindfully. Eating mindfully is the "How" component of digestion. We are not only digestion our food, we are digesting every impression involved in the experience. Eating in a stressful environment will impair our digestive functions because the stress hormones distract from the metabolic actions. If we eat when we are bored or sad, we are eating feelings of boredom and sadness. If we eat while we are distracted not only will we miss the goodness of the experience, we will also be more likely to miss the signals that inform us we are hungry or full.

Digestion starts with the senses. When we smell and see food we begin to salivate. This is the body's way of prepping for intake.

The entryway is significant. A lot happens in the mouth. As far as we are concerned, digestion begins in the mouth—not in the gut. Chewing your food thoroughly supports strong digestion, proper elimination, and portion control. Chewing also gives us a chance to savor and enjoy tastes. If we are eating at our desks, in the car, while carrying on assiduous conversations, or zoned out watching TV, we are not giving our food the chewing time it deserves. When we multitask blood is dispersed to various zones of the body to support multiple functions. If eating is part of a multi-tasking frenzy, the the blood and energy needed to convert food into usable fuel is not concentrated in the digestive organs. Our multiple efforts force the body to scatter our resources. Eating should be a unilateral event. Sit down, slow down, and chew thoroughly. Learn to really savor and appreciate your food. Allow eating to become a meditation of sorts.

> *"Fill your plate with the colors of the rainbow. What pleases the eye pleases the body as a whole."*
>
> **—Deepak Chopra**

Rhythms and Timing... What we eat matters, how we eat matters, and just as importantly—When we eat matters. Our digestive strength emulates the sun. The sun is lowest in the morning and night, and highest mid-day. Therefore, we should eat smaller meals in the morning and evening, and the biggest meal mid-day. When the sun is peaking, our digestive capacity is peaking. Also, food was designed to give us energy. When do we need energy? Mid-day. That is when we are thinking, doing things, accomplishing tasks, and being most active. We should eat a light balanced breakfast, a big lunch, and smaller dinner.

Our basal metabolic rate (how quickly we burn fuel) slows down as we prepare for rest, and drops again when we lie down. We convert energy differently at night verses the day. Plus, we do not need to stock a huge supply of energy before we sleep, because sleeping does not expend much energy. According to Ayurveda it is important to give time between meals so that we are not constantly layering food upon partially digested food matter. Piles on undigested food particles create Ama, or toxins in the body.

Intermitten Fasting…This concept has become very popular in recent years. Funny enough, the idea itself is thousands of years old. According to Ayurveda we should have a breakfast according to our hunger, a big lunch in the middle of the day, and a light dinner around sunset. Practically speaking, this means we have our fist meal around 8am and eat our last bite of food around 6 or 7pm. That gives us a 13-14 hour fasting window each day. This fasting period is a time of integration and rest. The GI doesn't need to be working all the time. If you're a Kapha, you likely are not hungry in the morning; so you'll probably eat lunch around noon and a light dinner around 5 or 6pm. This give you a 18 hour fasting window. You see fasting has always been in the design of health. In fact, that is why breakfast has it's name…its break-fast. The breaking of the fast. Industry has a remarkable way of selling us impressions, but the science reveals that Ayurveda is quite the trend setter.

> *"The mind and body are like parallel universes. Anything that happens in the mental universe must track in the physical one."*
>
> **—Deepak Chopra**

Poem…

Beautiful mothers
will you say to your daughters
You will always be spirit
You will always be truth
Yes, there is beauty in youth
but hard times will come
stand on your feet—laugh, act, rest, weep
Consider each challenge a stage for new strength
an ego sweep
ride the wrinkles of time
allow life to earn you your lines
Don't cover them up
they are the accolades of well lived days
Spend time with your soul
do not knock yourself down
save yourself from the suffering of comparison.
be kind
be gracious
be generous
be daring

and especially to those who are not…

be markedly caring

Just when you think it can not get worse

it just might

but just when you think it can not get better—it will—it will do that too

My beautiful daughter, you will always be spirit, you will always be truth. Do not waste your youth trying to make yourself any better, any more, or any different than you are now because one day you'll turn around to find that now has not moved, or it moved with you. You could not evade it, so for heavens sake, do not escape it. Wrap your loving arms around the caracal of life. It is on your team. My daughter, just believe.

CHAPTER THIRTEEN

Your Fork and Your Psychology

"If you are what you eat, you might as well eat something good."

—Ratatouille

THE MIND-BODY CONNECTION to food... How Food Effects Our Psychology: We know the constitutions of the mind-body: Vata, Pitta and Kapha, but there is more. In addition to our mind-body constitutions, we have emotional constitutions as well. Our psychological constitutions are mental and emotional traits characterized under the three names: Sattva, Rajas, and Tamas. Similar to the mind-body constitution, it is desirable to keep our physiological constitution in a state of equilibrium. As an extension of the Doshas, the principles are not dissimilar. We all have all three within us, and the three are malleable—vulnerable to fluctuations in accordance to our situations, relationships, food and lifestyle. **Rajas** is the energy that wakes us up in the morning. It is a sprightly and motivated energy that initiates movement. Too much Rajas can lead to a climate of over work, hyper movements, rapid-fire thoughts, competition, and judgement. This sounds similar to Pitta Dosha, which is why Pittas have a proclivity to have excess Rajas or to be more Rajastic. **Tamas** is the opposite. Tamas is the energy that puts us to sleep at night. This energy is heavy, dull, and slow. We need this energy to relax and unwind, but too much Tamas can lead to inertia and even depression. The qualities of Tamas are similar to some Kapha qualities, which is why Kaphas can easily become Tamastic. **Sattva.** The desirable place in the middle of the opposite ends of the energetic spectrum is called—Sattva. Purity, truth, and contentment live within Sattva. Cultivating Sattva helps us to manage stress and feel calm. We we are Sattvic we move through our days with creatively, inspiration, and serenity. Because we feel so peaceful, Sattva gives us a buffer to impending stresses and distractions that throughout the day. There are multiple ways to cultivate this truthful, pure, and content state. Nature is a wonderful way to promote Sattva, therefor eating natural food intrinsically promotes Sattva.

Eating Sattvic foods is a way to insert balance into your life three times a day. Sattvic foods are whole foods. Seasonal fruits, vegetables, grains, nuts, seeds, ghee and honey. Processed foods that have been refined, fortified, spritzed with pesticides, injected with antibiotics, saturated in chemicals, or altered in factories are not Sattvic. 90% of the food on our grocery store shelves are not Sattvic. The lessons we have already integrated can be superimposed here. Buying organic, shopping at farmers markets, choosing items from the parameters of the market or growing your own food will help ensure that your food is fresh and Sattvic in nature. The way the food is prepared is important. Food should not be cooked or eaten in a hurry, while angry, mindlessly or without gratitude because the heartbeat of Sattva is patient, joyous, mindful, and grateful. As we now appreciate, we are not only what we eat—but also how we eat. Eating slowly in a peaceful environment will increase Sattva.

Prana and Sattva go hand and hand. Their relationship is symbiotic. Whole foods are full of Prana and remind us of our Sattvic nature. Stimulating substances like coffee, caffeine, alcohol, citrus juices, garlic, onions and hot peppers increase Rajas. These foods can make us aggressive, irritable, and competitive. They are incredibly acidic and heating. Over indulgence in heating/acidic/stimulating foods will make us feel like we have been in a hot tub too long. We will feel irritable and itchy to get out. If we ca not get out, we can become frustrated and aggressive. So, avoid an over consumption of Rajastic foods because they move us away from Sattva. On the other side: too many heavy foods like dairy, sugar, wheat, and meat can make us feel cloudy, dull, and heavy. Dead foods or foods that are left over, stale, processed, microwaved, void of taste, fried or burnt have a similar effect. These foods have minimal Prana, so we will feel lifeless after eating them. Eating too much, too late, or while upset can lead to Tamas as well. This would be like sitting in a mud bath for too long. Eventually we would just feel heavy and stuck, and unable to move. To avoid feeling Tamastic, avoid processed/nuked/heavy/dead foods.

Sattvic food are not extreme in tastes, therefore we can bypass extreme emotions or mood swings by eating Sattvic foods. By becoming Sattvic we seamlessly bend towards balancing our Doshas and aligning our 5 elements. This is because whole foods tend to carry the correct combinations of elements and are not extreme in taste. Each of the six tastes spur a mental implication. For example: sweet will illicit devotion but greed in excess. Sour creates desire but too much leads to envy. Salty adds a zest to life, but too much could propel hedonism. Pungent tastes is stimulating, but causes anger in excess. Bitter helps us face reality, but leads to feeling chronically dissatisfied if consumed in excess. And astringent tastes helps us tap into introspection, but can lead to loneliness and anxiety in excess.

By having a little of each taste in each meal, not only will our physical bodies feel nourished, but our hearts and minds reap the reward as well. Extreme tastes like really spicy (hot sauce), or super sweet (candy) are not Sattvic. Whereas Kitchari for example is perfectly Sattvic. Kitchari one of Ayurveda's premier balancing foods because the rice is sweet, the beans are astringent, the turmeric is bitter, a pinch of salt and pepper is added to achieve salty and pungent—and the post digestive effect is sour—rounding us out with all six tastes. To eat a balanced meal in a peaceful environment in the company of good friends will surely promote your most pleasant mental disposition, Sattva.

PAUSE FOR AFFIRMATION

"I am consuming Sattvic foods to promote my sense of peace and clarity."

Sweet tastes have the primordial correlation to being soothed and put to ease. Breast milk is sweet and it was, for most of us, the first thing we tasted. We're wired to associate sweet tastes to the feeling of being nurtured and cared for. That's why when we're stressed or overwhelmed, we often crave sweets. We want to be reminded that we're safe and everything's going to be okay. Sweet and survival are in our hardwiring. You can substitute artificial or heavy sweet tastes for Golden Milk if you're stressed. You can even add stevia or honey. You will have the response of being nurtured without having to consume the negative side effects that accompany sugary items.

Ayurvedic Food is not just Indian food, and all Indian food is not Ayurvedic. I often have clients say to me, "I want to eat Ayurvedic food, but I do not like the taste of Indian food." As we have illustrated that the principles and applications of Ayurvedic nutrition are not limited to eating Indian food, loving curry, and drinking chai tea. Eating Ayurvedically means that we apply the fundamental laws of balance to nourish ourselves. This means listening to your body, noticing the qualities of food and the qualities in your body and applying the rule of opposites to create balance. Eating Ayurvedically means you are making an effort to nourish yourself with whole foods and a variety of tastes and textures so that you can achieve balance, and feel the way you want to feel. Eating Ayurvedically means that you are present and mindful when you are eating. Ayurvedic food has nothing to do with cultural cuisine. Ayurvedic food has everything to do with mindful awareness. We may not have a taste for curry just yet, but we certainly have an appetite for feeling our best.

"Seems you can not outsmart mother nature."

—Mark Hyman

CHAPTER FOURTEEN

Ama and Detoxifying

"The best way to detoxify is to stop putting toxic things in the body, and depend upon its own mechanisms."

—Andrew Weil

AMA... AMA IS the Ayurveda term for toxins, sludge, gunk and waste that block our channels and suppress our functions. Undigested thoughts, experiences, and emotions create mental Ama, whereas undigested food creates physical Ama. Ama weakens our metabolism and impairs on the natural flow of energy throughout the body. Ama can be responsible for lethargy, depression, arthritis, constipation, headaches, and acne to name a few.

Eating at right times, giving space between meals, eating for your constitution and keeping your digestive fire strong are the best ways to prevent Ama. Drinking ginger tea with a pinch of black pepper or an herb called Trikatu (a combination of indian long pepper, black pepper and ginger) will help burn away

Ama and spark your digestive fire. Using digestive spices will help you detoxify Ama and prevent future build up. Drinking Detox and Replenish Tea helps mitigate and remove Ama.

Incompatibles. Ayurveda understands that some foods just do not agree with each other. Combining certain foods can create a combative atmosphere in the gut. This conflict can create indigestion and Ama. The Ancient texts set the following guidelines:

» Beans should not be eaten with fruit, cheese, eggs fish, milk or yogurt. (Such as in a burrito)

» Eggs should not be eaten with fruit (especially melons), beans, cheese, fish, meat or dairy. (Such as an omelette)

» Fruit should not be eaten with other food unless it is cooked.

» Honey should not be eaten with equal parts ghee.

» Lemon should not be eaten with cucumbers, dairy or tomatoes.

» Melons should be eaten alone. (You might recall a few gassy picnics because of this one.)

» Nightshades (potatoes, eggplants, tomatoes, chilis and sweet bell peppers) should not be eaten with dairy. (Eggplant parmesan anyone?)

» Radishes should not be eaten with bananas, dairy or raisins.

» Yogurt should not be eaten with fruit, cheese, fish, meat or nightshades. (No more parfaits.)

I realize some of these sound like hideous combinations that you would never dream of putting together anyway, but some of these combinations are popular in our culture. Look at the parfait. Fruit and dairy. This is not good because the fruit is light and easy to digest, while the dairy is hard to digest. One has to wait its turn. While waiting, the dairy will curdle and the fruit will ferment. This creates gas, bloating and toxemia. Salads with fruits, bacon and eggs, tomatoes with mozzarella cheese, eggs with cheese, black bean and queso quesadillas or tacos, other common combos that create indigestion and Ama.

Your ability to handle incompatible food combinations relates to your digestive strength. If your Agni is strong, you might occasionally eat these items without discomfort, but if your Agni is weak you are more likely to experience negative reactions. For the same reason, combing raw foods with cooked foods in the same meal can wreak havoc because the cooked foods are already partially broken down, but the raw food requires more effort to break down in the body. Fruit is considered "pre-digested," meaning it is so easy to breakdown that in theory—it can pass from mouth to elimination in less than an hour. Because of this, fruit should be eaten alone as a snack or 30-45 minutes before your meal or two-three hours after your meal. This way the fruit will not have to wait its turn to digest with the rest of the meal.

How Sleep Affects your Metabolism. Sleep is a time to reboot. Our metabolic hormones regenerate while we are asleep. If we get less than 6-8 hours of sleep our hormones will be very disoriented. Erratic sleep patterns can affect the functions of storing carbohydrates and regulating leptin and ghrelin, the two hormones that are responsible for appetite control. Without proper sleep it is hard to decipher when we are hungry and when we are full. Chronic sleep deprivation can lead to false cravings and higher body mass index (a Kapha imbalance). Sometimes when we are tired, we will reach for a quick fix like caffeine, alcohol, or food. When there is a lack of proper rest no amount of sugary, salty snacks will suffice. What we need is sleep. We have all experienced how sleep impacts of energy and moods. Keep in mind that sleep also effects your metabolism.

How Stress Impacts Your Metabolism. Stress and anxiety can lead to nervous eating habits. When we are stressed we release a hormone called cortisol. Cortisol is a "flight or fight" hormone released by the adrenals. It's normal to release cortisol throughout the day, but when we are chronically stressed our levels stay high the cortisol takes up residency in the but, hips, thighs and waist. This leads to insulin resistance and increased inflammation and weight gain (Kapha and Pitta disorders). Visceral fat or fat in the organs is more hazardous to our health. It is important to befriend meditation and self-care routines to help keep stress levels at a minimum.

Eat Seasonally. Eat what is in season. A plentiful seasonal harvest is God's way of saying, "Go on, eat this now." Nature has an intelligence and finesse that we cannot replicate. Is something is seasonally grown in our environment, it is intended to be consumed to create balance. For example, coconuts are bountiful in the summer months in tropical environments because they will cool the body (balance Pitta). Hearty root vegetables are plentiful in the fall in the cold climates because they will warm and ground the body (balance Vata). Eat as the season would dictate.

General Nutritional Guidelines That Apply To All Three Doshas...

Encourage:

Whole grains, seasonal fruits, seasonal vegetables, nuts/seeds, (lesser amounts) organic chicken, fish, ghee/coconut oil, olive oil, and honey.

Avoid:

Processed/artificial foods. Foods that are fried, burnt, stale or microwaved. Excess sodium (salt), sugar, oil and red meat (saturated fat). Copious amounts of coffee and alcohol (Pitta types should highlight this).

> *"With every drop of water you drink, every breath you take, you're connected to the sea. No matter where on earth you live."*
>
> **—Sylvia Earle**

Fluids. What we drink is as critical to our health as what we eat. Eliminating sports drinks and sodas is the first call to action. Theses drinks are inundated with chemicals. Zero calorie waters and diet drinks are no better, in fact maybe worse. Aspartame, and like chemicals found in diet drinks lead to nervousness, neurological and autoimmune disorders. Plus, they can feed addictions and induce false cravings. Just because something does not have calories, does not mean it is good for you. Cocaine is calorie free but it sure is heck will not make you healthier. If you drink a lot of coffee you may want to cut back, (especially Vatas because of nervousness and Pittas because of acidity). One or two cups a day is suitable unless you suffer from ulcers, colitis, anxiety, tremors, or insomnia. If you have trouble sleeping, do not drink caffeine after 3pm. Note what you are putting in your coffee. Coffee shops often pump syrups of sugar and chemicals into our mystery cups of goodness. Opt for almond milk and sugar in the raw instead. Sprinkling a pinch of cardamom in your coffee will help neutralize the effects of acid and caffeine. If you drink alcohol, note that wine and beer are the least irritating. However beer will increase Kapha Dosha. Hard liquors really exasperate Pitta Dosha because their ultra heating. Vodka with soda water and mint or cilantro, (like a mojito) will be less abrasive to your stomach lining than dark liquors. Careful not to combine the liquor with sugary mixers like soda or juice. This will increase your risk for dehydration, weight gain and hangovers. If you are going out for a night on the town or celebrating with friends, drink a glass of water between each alcoholic beverage to minimize dehydration and over consumption. We are not aiming to be perfect. Imbalances, fumbles and woes are staples of life. On your birthday, enjoy your birthday cake! 21st birthday? Go out with your friends and celebrate! Girls night—have a glass of wine and giggle until your soul smiles! We are not robots, but if you feel you have grown dependent on food or alcohol as a coping mechanism or vice—look deeply. The alcohol or food are not the culprits. What is actually bothering you? Getting to the heart of the issue will receive you from masking what needs to be healed. Healing happens from a place of awareness.

Make sure you are drinking enough water. Imbalances such as headache, constipation, bloating, PMS, scanty sweat and urine, memory loss, poor concentration, uncontrollable hunger, cravings, and fatigue can be do to dehydration. Vatas need the most water because of their dry quality. Pittas will usually feel thirsty, so that should prompt drinking, while Kaphas require less water because water is already part of their elemental makeup. In general, we should all drink about 8 glasses of water a day. If you sweat a lot, live in a dry climate or drink diuretics like coffee you should replenish with more water. Always drink your water warm or room temp, never cold. As we mentioned, cold water suppresses the digestive fire —promoting gas, bloating and indigestion, constricts the channels and coagulates fat.

> *"Drinking water is like taking a shower on the inside of your body."*
>
> **—Unknown**

Teas are a wonderful way to get fluids into the body: Digestive Tea is good for everyone: Take equal parts ¼ tsp powdered ginger, whole fennel seeds, whole cumin seeds and whole coriander pods and combine in hot water. (see appendix for resources on an organic pre-made version by wellBlends). Allow it to steep for 3-5 minutes and enjoy. You can have this tea up to three times a day. It's perfect with or in between meals. Kaphas do well with a warming tea. Take a pinch of cinnamon, a pinch of ginger powder and a pinch of clove powder and combine the spices with one cup of hot water. All the water to infuse for 3-5 minutes and then enjoy.

CHAPTER FIFTEEN

Modern Dilemmas and Considerations

"Begin to see yourself as a soul with a body, rather than a body with a soul."

—Wayne Dyer

MODERN DILEMMAS. Chemicals-Chemicals have become part of our cultural atmosphere. We cannot scare ourselves into a sterilized room just because we are afraid of chemicals, but we can make conscious decisions to avoid them when possible. As we now know eating whole foods will help you reduce your exposure to chemicals. Eating organic whole foods will safeguard you even more. If you want to stop eating chemicals, avoiding processed foods is imperative. There are foods on our shelves that are literally banned in other countries thanks to their obvious and proven dangers. Artificial food dye found in cereals, macaroni and cheese, sports drinks, candy, cheese and cake mixes. Olestra, found in potato chips, french fries and corn chips. Brominated vegetable oil, found in sports drinks and citrus sodas. Potassium bromate, found in wraps, rolls, bread crumbs, bagels and breads. Azodicabonamide, found in breads, frozen dinners, boxed pastas and packaged baked goods. BHA and BHT, found in cereal, nut mixes, gum, butter, meat and dehydrated potatoes. Synthetic growth hormones, found in milk and dairy products. And arsenic, found in poultry. These common chemicals stock are grocery store shelves and line our pantries without our knowing. They can cause cancer, diabetes, organ failure, neurological imbalances, and autoimmune disease to name a few. By checking labels and eating whole foods, you can protect yourself and your family.

Dairy. Shedding light on a big misconception...I don't think being a vegetarian, pescetarian, starburstarian or any kind of "terian" is the answer. We are unique ever evolving beings, in such I do not identify with a one-size fits all approach to food. On average we make close to 200 decision regarding food ever single day. Do I want fish or chicken? Grilled or fried? Blacked on plain? Can you pass the salt? Is there MSG in that? Want fries with that? Want an extra shot of espresso in that? Boggling! Studies show that we are conscious of a mere 15% of food based decisions we face on a daily basis. Personally, I eat mostly plants. I do not eat dairy. No milk, no cheese, no yogurt—nada. Dairy creates cellular inflammation and mucus. Dairy is a contributing factor for skin conditions, digestive disorders, hormonal imbalances and weakened immune functions. Personally ditching dairy was a simple habit to kick because I never had an affinity for it anyway. I swapped milk for almond milk and called it a day. With that said, I know many friends who have a deep affection for their beloved dairy companions. In that case, play with reducing your consumption. Flirt with the idea of replacing cheese and crackers for hummus with crackers. You will get the same texture without the negative side effects. If you are shaking your pretty little head thinking, 'No way Jose', swap cows cheese for goats cheese. It's easier to digest and reeks less havoc. Allow this perspective to wash over you... Humans are the only creatures who drink the milk of another creature. Baby cows drink their mamas milk to gain hundreds of pounds in their first year of life. Why are we drinking it? Beats me. Well, I have one idea. Remember the ads, "Got milk?" The most gorgeous and handsome faces in Hollywood have been posing this question while wearing milk mustaches for decades. The FDA food pyramid sensationalizes dairy. Dairy is packaged with bold claims to protect your bones and make you big and strong. While these slogans may be attractive, they are false. The first question people ask when they learn I don't consume dairy is, "Well then how do you get enough calcium?" Great question. Dairy actually causes our bones to leech calcium because it is hyper acidic. The calcium from our bones neutralizes the acids from milk (and meat). Leafy greens and lentils are a far better source of calcium—plus they are alkaline. Your bones will benefit from ditching dairy. The common misconception is credited to years of misleading information and marketing. And to layer onto that, we should experience more caution now than ever because our current model for dairy farming involves antibiotics, hormone and steroid injections—as well as a notable environmental impact. The hormone IGF or insulin-like growth factor mimics the effects of human growth hormones in negative ways. These anabolic hormones are associated with increase risks of prostate, breast cancer, and tumors. According to Ayurveda, the sweet taste of milk gives it a building effect—building excess tissues. Any excess is defined as a Kapha imbalance. Kapha imbalances are directly related to heaviness, weight gain and lethargy. If you experience these symptoms you have added motivation to eliminate dairy from your diet. Kale, collard greens, spinach, kelp and soybeans top the list for calcium rich plant foods. These foods are also packed with anti-oxidants, anti-inflammatory properties and they have a lightening (or catabolic) effect on the body and mind. These are better options. At the end of the day, we are all doing the best we can. Eating dairy is clearly not criminal, but if you have digestive, hormonal or skin imbalances skip the dairy and see how you feel. Feeling better will instantly reinforce your positive decision, and will surely motivate you to continue down your bright and healthy path. At the height of Arnold Schwarzeneggers weight lifting career he was asked if he drinks milk. His answer..."Milk is for babies."

Vegetarianism. Becoming a vegetarian is not everyone's cup of tea, and to be healthy—it is not necessary. If you are going to eat meat choose free range/grass fed/ organic chicken and beef. If you eat fish, choose wild fish or organically farmed fish to avoid chemicals. Try not to eat large fish like marlin, tuna, king mackerel, and swordfish more than once or twice a week because bigger fish that are higher up the food chain contain bigger amounts of mercury. Avoid processed sausages and deli meats that are laden with chemicals, preservatives, and additives. Everyone should reduce their consumption of red meat as it leads to heart disease, high cholesterol, type 2 diabetes, and obesity. If you are interested in becoming a vegetarian but are concerned about meeting your protein requirements, fear not. Currently, Americans eat more protein than ever and we are no stronger, smarter or healthier because of it. Worldwide, meat consumption doubled between 1950 and 2009. The average person eats about one quarter pound of animal meat a day. If this trend continues, by 2050 we will be eating two-thirds more animal protein than we are today. That takes a toll on our planet and our digestive organs. We get plenty of protein from vegetables, beans, eggs, soy and grains. Ayurveda is not suggesting that we all become vegetarians, but for our personal health and global health, it would be advantageous to reduce our consumption of animal protein.

> *"Nothing will benefit health and increase the chances for survival on earth as the evolution of a vegetarian diet."*
>
> **—Einstein**

Environmental Impact: Raising animals requires a large amount of energy. It takes about 25 hundred gallons of water to produce one pound of beef versus 25 gallons of water to produce one pound of wheat. Our current consumption is draining aquifers around the world. 40% of our water is used to irrigate crops that feed our livestock. To give some context on what a large quantity that really is, only 13% is used for domestic purposes such as showering, flushing toilets, doing laundry, washing cars, and watering our lawns. Other environmental impacts include the depletion of fossil fuels and topsoil, pollution of the water and air from cow manure and urine (2.7 trillion pounds of manure each year), deforestation of the rainforest to create space to herd fast-food beef and methane gas given off from livestock. This gas traps heat in the atmosphere. Theoretically, reducing our meat consumption could reduce the speed of global warming. I am not proselytizing that we all stop eating meat, but for the sake of our health and environment; reducing our meat consumption is a smart move.

"Get people back in the kitchen and combat the trend toward processed and fast food."

—Dr. Andrew Weil

Time Management and Prep. Convenience has become a major selling point in our decision making processes. By taking the time to plan and prep meals and meal ideas you will be less likely to fall into the slippery trap of always grabbing, "What's convenient." It is possible to organize your eating routine in such a way that eating freshly made meals actually becomes convenient. Orchestrating your meals is can be simple and is notably valuable whether it's for you or your entire family. As we discussed, choose a few staple items and make them in bulk.

Pre-wash and cut all your favorite veggies so you can quickly and easily grab them to stir fry, roast or grill. Bake or Grill chicken or fish in bulk a couple times a week. You can play with these items creatively. Fresh ingredients translate into endless varieties of cuisine. Sauté in coconut milk and curry for thai, soy sauce for Chinese, drizzle with olive oil and sprinkle with oregano for Italian, use ghee and spiced (curry) for Indian, sauté with chili and onion and top with salsa for Mexican. Being playful with spices creates diversity and dimension. Utilize the crock pot for soups and chilies. Keep washed and fresh fruits in the fridge or on the counter. Have your go to breakfast like oatmeal with ghee and cinnamon, baked fruit drizzled with balsamic and sprinkled with cardamom or a quick omelet with with turmeric and black pepper. Eating well does not need to be complicated. Once you get in the rhythm, it will feel second nature.

"One can not think well, love well, sleep well is one is not dined well."

—Virgina Woolf

Eating Out. Eating out can be fun and the positive social influence can boost our emotional wellbeing. But for our health eating out should be a treat, not the norm. If you can find a local restaurant that serves dishes made from organic ingredients, excellent! Many restaurants nowadays offer plenty of healthy options. As we have learned not be fooled by labels like "veggie burger," "gluten free," "fat free" and the like. These items are typically highly processed. Be skillful. Choose steamed or sautéed veggies, a baked sweet potato, brown rice, wild rice or quinoa and baked or grilled chicken or fish. If you order a salad, choose oil and vinegar or balsamic over a heavy dressing that may be loaded with sodium, high fructose corn syrup and sugar. Combine all the information you have gathered with your health savvy common sense and make the best decision. I usually check the menu online before I go. Don't be bashful about asking the server to make adjustments for you. The restaurant industry is service driven, they want to please the customer. Plus, when enough of us speak up, more healthy options appear.

Practice: *If you currently drink cold fluids, this week swap all of your cold beverages for warm versions. Incorporate hot teas and plenty of room temperature or warm water. Notice how the temperature of the fluids benefits the strength of your Agni, your ability to comfortably digest food, and helps you prevent Ama within the GI.*

CHAPTER SIXTEEN

Meal Plans and Recipes

> *"A recipe has no soul. You as the cook must bring the soul to the recipe."*
>
> **—Thomas Keller**

USE SPICES. We use spices to boost our Agni (digestive fire), reduce toxins, increase the absorption and assimilation of nutrients, improve circulation, enhance immunity, alleviate gas and bloating, illuminate lethargy and modulate weight to name a few. We look at nutrition through the lens of elements (space, air, fire, water and earth), qualities (light, heavy, cold, hot, moist, dry, etc.) and tastes (sweet, sour, salty, pungent, bitter and astringent.)

Everything we consume is built upon these characteristics, and elicits a correlating response in the body. We use the philosophy that, "Like Increases Like" and "Opposites Create Balance". For example, if someone is always hot, suffers from migraines, occasionally gets skin rashes and angers easily—they have excess heat in the body. This person will want to use cooling spices like coriander and fennel to create balance. If another person is cold, heavy, and lethargic they will benefit from light/heating spices like ginger and cayenne pepper. Spices can be used to balance each Dosha, improve digestion and create homeostasis. These spices can be added to freshly prepared meals and even teas. The various mixtures may include, but are not limited to: turmeric, cumin, coriander, fennel, ginger, cinnamon, cardamom, clove, black pepper, salt, cayenne and asafetida (hing).

» Turmeric—Anti-oxidant, anti-inflammatory. Fights free radicals, slows process of aging, cleanses blood and detoxifies the liver.

» Ginger—Increases Agni. Reduces inflammation. Cures nausea.

» Cumin—Detoxifies the liver and kidneys. Aids in nutrient absorption.

» Fennel—Packed with trace minerals. Helps detox excess fat from tissues. Works as a natural apposite suppressant.

» Coriander—Alleviates gas and bloating. Cools the body.

» Cinnamon—Helps to regulate glucose levels and promotes optimal circulation.

» Cayenne Pepper—Burns toxins, clears excess phlegm and sparks Agni.

» Himalayan Salt—Full of trace minerals, helps regulate blood volume, lowers blood pressure and slows muscle contractions.

» Nutmeg—Works as a mild sedative to calm the nervous system.

» Black Pepper—Boost Agni, clears mucus and phlegm.

Medicinal Uses for Spices

> *"When we develop reverence for food and the miracle of transformation internet in it, just the simple act of eating creates a ritual of celebration."*
>
> **—Deepak Chopra**

What is Ghee? Ghee is a popular form of fat used for cooking and flavoring food. It is also used as a carrier to get Ayurvedic medicines into the body. Ghee is clarified butter. It is made from free-range, grass fed cows. The organic, unsalted butter is prepared into ghee by simmering the butter which is churned from cream. Once the butter is melted and the animal (dairy) lipids are separated from the pure fats, the impurities from the surface are skimmed off and discarded, and the clear liquid fat is poured into a clean jar for use. The solid residue from impure fats at the bottom of the pot are also thrown out. All that is left in the process of making ghee is a healthy form of fat that is similar in nutrition to coconut oil. Ghee is considered vegan because the animal properties have been cooked out and skimmed off. Ghee does not raise your cholesterol as much as regular butter.

It promotes a balanced agni, and is a clean source of fat for the body. It is also a sattvic food. Ghee is considered healing and sacred. In India, ghee is offered to the gods in temples in times of worship.

Meal Plans and Recipes. I would encourage you to just get in the kitchen with simple fresh ingredients and spices. The good news is when you are playing with quality ingredients, the chances of your creation being good are in your favor. I personally live out of my wok. I stir-fry everything. I included a few fun and easy recipes, but my list is not exhaustive. Be resourceful and take advantage of the endless array of tools and inspiration at your fingertips. While the internet is not totally reliable for health advice, it is bursting with brilliant recipes and ideas.The meal plans are not intended to be strictly followed, rather they are exemplary of appropriate ways to nourish each Dosha. The meal plans are templates to give you a basic structure on how to get started. If eating home cooked meals every day sounds like a long shot, just start slow. Perhaps you can dabble with one home cooked meal a day and build from there. Remember, sustainable shifts need to be practical and pleasant. In time, these principles will become so ingrained in you that you will find yourself intuitively applying them anytime you order from a menu, peruse a buffet line or celebrate with friends over a good meal.

"The most indispensable ingredient of all good home cooking: love those you are cooking for."

—Sophia Loren

VATA MEAL PLAN:

This plan is appropriate for a Vata constitution or someone with a Vata body type imbalance. Start your day with a glass of warm water.

Breakfast Ideas:

(Avoid cold and dry breakfast cereals.)

- » Egg omelette with spinach turmeric and black pepper.
- » Oatmeal with 1 tsp. of ghee, 1 tsp. cinnamon, and 1 tbs. of flaxseed powder. Can add raisins and walnuts.
- » Sweet potato, with warm organic applesauce and cinnamon. Drizzle with ghee.
- » Baked apple (slice and bake for 10 minutes), drizzle with balsamic vinegar and add a dash of cardamom powder.

Avoid coffee because of the stimulation factor, but if you drink coffee—avoid syrups or flavored creamers. Use almond milk or coconut milk and a dash of cardamom.

Lunch Ideas:

(Avoid raw: especially in the fall and winter)

- » Sweet potato, asparagus or other green veggies with a piece of organic chicken or wild fish.

  **You can substitute chicken or fish with 1 tbs of flaxseed powder, 1 tbs. of nutritional yeast, 2 eggs or a handful of nuts and seeds.*

» Mediterranean bowl: warm basmati rice, sliced assorted olives, chickpeas soaked in olive oil, and parsley.

Dinner Ideas:

» Thai snow pea curry: snow peas and carrots and diced tofu sautéed in coconut oil with 1 tbs. of curry powder. Serve with basmati rice cooked with a dash of turmeric and several cardamom pods.

» Spaghetti squash, sautéed spinach cooked in ghee or sesame oil with wild rice and pine nuts.

» Lentils, quinoa, and green beans cooked in ghee and garlic.

» Brussels sprouts baked with slice grapes, olive oil, a couple cloves of garlic, oregano, basil and thyme. Bake at 350 degrees for 20 minutes. Serve with ½-1 cup of quinoa or basmati rice.

» Grilled zucchini and onions with collard greens sautéed in ghee and garlic powder or basil. Add a dash of Agni kindling spice mix and 1 tbs of flaxseed powder or nutritional yeast for protein.

The Go To: *(staple choices)*

Sautéed broccoli and cauliflower. Cooked in ghee or coconut oil with a generous dash of Agni kindling spices. Add eggs, seeds or flaxseed powder for protein. Fill your plate and enjoy!

Order up! *(from a menu)*

Hearty soups: chili, squash and beans are great!

Snacks: Carrot or Date Balls (see recipe) dates, avocados, nuts, seeds, baked fruit (apple/pear) with ghee and cinnamon.

Sip: ginger, cumin, fennel and coriander tea. Seep ½ tsp in hot water for 5 minutes. (see appendix for pre-made blend) Warm water, chamomile, ginger, raspberry or eucalyptus tea.

Spice mix: hing, turmeric, ginger, coriander, cumin, fennel, fenugreek and black pepper. Can use salt and cayenne. (see appendix B for "Agni" spice blend)

Avoid: white sugar, caffeine, and alcohol.

In Your Fridge: Pre-baked sweet potatoes, a Tupperware of quinoa or basmati rice, precut veggies (zucchini, onions, broccoli, cauliflower, carrots, asparagus and spinach), a Tupperware of red lentils or mung beans, avocados, and pre-washed mangoes, strawberries and papaya.

In your pantry: Nuts, seeds, oats, ghee, coconut oil and herbal teas.

> *"Learn how to cook, try new recipes, learn from your mistakes, be fearless and above all have fun."*
>
> **—Julia Child**

PITTA MEAL PLAN:

This plan is appropriate for a Pitta constitution or someone with a Pitta body type imbalance. Start your day with a glass of warm water. If you have hyperacidity add a slice of lemon.

Breakfast Ideas:

» Egg white omelette with kale (any leafy green), turmeric and black pepper.

» Oatmeal with 1 tsp. of coconut oil, 1 tsp. cinnamon, and 1 tbs. of flaxseed powder.

» Carrot and Oat Balls (see recipe below)

» Raw granola (avoid the highly processed box variations) with almond milk.

If you drink coffee, avoid syrups or flavored creamers. Use almond milk or coconut milk and a dash of cardamom.

Lunch ideas:

» Kale salad: kale, sliced almonds, dried cranberries, olive oil, salt and pepper with a squeeze of lemon.

» Carrots with hummus, sautéed bitter greens cooked in coconut oil, turmeric and ginger with a cup of lentils or piece of organic chicken or freshwater fish.

» Arugula with sliced avocado, cucumber, olives, sunflower seeds and dates. Drizzle with olive oil, use fresh cilantro or a dash of dried basil.

- Sweet potato, asparagus or other green veggies with a piece of organic chicken or wild fish.

**can substitute chicken or fish with 1 tbs of flaxseed powder, 1 tbs of nutritional yeast, 2 eggs (whites are cooling) or a handful of sunflower or pumpkin seeds.*

Dinner Ideas:

- Thai kale: kale and chickpeas sautéed in coconut milk with a tbs of curry powder. Serve alone or with basmati rice cooked with a dash of turmeric and several cardamom pods.
- Mediterranean plate: olives, cucumbers, a slice of tomato with cilantro or mint with 1 sliced avocado.
- Lentils, quinoa and greens cooked with Agni spices and ghee.
- Brussels sprouts baked with slice grapes, olive oil, a couple cloves of garlic, oregano, basil and thyme. Bake at 350 degrees for 20 minutes. Serve with ½-1 cup of quinoa or
- Grilled bell peppers and mushrooms with collard greens sautéed in ghee or coconut oil. Add a dash of your spice mix and 1 tbs of flaxseed powder or nutritional yeast for protein.
- Couscous with peas cooked with ghee turmeric and ginger.
- Nutritious Wrap: cucumber, parsley, black olives, sprouts, sweet peppers and hummus in a lentil wrap.

The Go To: *(staples)*

Sautéed broccoli and cauliflower. Cooked in ghee or coconut oil with a generous dash of Agni kindling spices. Add eggs or flax seed for protein. Fill your plate and enjoy!

Snacks: carrots, celery, apples, pears, dates, cranberries, cucumbers, watermelon and coconut (shredded or fresh).

Sip: ginger, cumin,fennel and coriander tea. Seep ½ tsp in hot water for 5 minutes (Detox and Replenish Tea by Wellblends) Room temp water. Coconut water (during the summer), mint, chamomile or raspberry tea.

Indian spice mix: turmeric, ginger, coriander, cumin, fennel, fenugreek and black pepper. Cilantro is great! (See appendix B for "Agni" spice blend)

Avoid: citrus juice, alcohol and coffee in excess.

In Your Fridge: Pre-baked sweet potatoes, a Tupperware of quinoa, couscous or basmati rice, organic egg whites, pre-cut and washed veggies (kale, broccoli, cauliflower, carrots and Brussels sprouts and cucumbers), pre-soaked chickpeas, pre-washed apples, pears watermelon and sweet berries. Pre-baked chicken and freshwater fish.

In Your Pantry: Oats, basmati rice, dried dates, dried coconut shavings, ghee, coconut oil and herbal tea.

> *"The only real stumbling block is fear of failure. In cooking you've got to have a what-the-hell attitude."*
>
> **—Julia Child**

KAPHA MEAL PLANS:

This plan is appropriate for a Kapha constitution or someone with a Kapha body type imbalance. Start your day with warm water with lemon or ginger tea.

Breakfast Ideas:

» Keep it light. A combination of apples, berries, cherries, persimmons, pomegranates and cranberries.

» Puffed cereal (organic, made with minimal ingredients/additives and processing) with almond milk and cinnamon.

» Cooked cereal: barley or buckwheat with cinnamon.

» Savory: Quinoa with sautéed onions, leafy greens or peas. Add turmeric, ginger and black pepper.

If you drink coffee: Avoid dairy, syrups or flavored creamers. Use almond milk and a dash of cardamom powder.

Lunch Ideas:

» Kale salad: kale, dried cranberries and a few pumpkin seeds with sunflower oil, pepper and squeeze of lemon.

» Grilled onions, bell peppers and Brussels sprouts sprinkled with oregano, rosemary and basil with quinoa.

» Sautéed collard greens cooked in ghee and garlic with sliced tomatoes and basil or mint served with a piece of organic chicken or freshwater fish.

**Can substitute chicken or fish with 1 tsp nutritional yeast, 1 cup cooked beans/ lentils or a small handful of pumpkin, sunflower or chia seeds for protein.*

» Bake mushrooms, artichokes and asparagus in sunflower oil and oregano serve with freshwater fish, organic chicken or a cup of black beans with black pepper.

» Mustard or dandelion greens and chickpeas sautéed in a little coconut milk (just enough for moisture. Not drowning in it) and plenty of curry powder. Serve with ½-1 cup of millet cooked with 1 tsp of turmeric and a few cardamom pods.

Dinner Ideas:

This is the lightest meal.

Soups:

» Veggies, cabbage, black bean, lentil, broth based. No hearty/creamy soups.

» Arugula salad with sliced veggies and balsamic vinegar.

» 2 eggs, sliced tomato and fresh basil.

- Grilled chicken or fish with sautéed greens (green beans, collard/dandelion greens, kale or spinach) cooked in a little ghee or sunflower oil with garlic or Indian spice mix (see below)
- Sliced avocado, with carrots and hummus. Sip on warm broth (chicken or vegetable).
- Mexican wrap: black beans, spinach, salsa, hot peppers, cilantro and sprouts in an organic rice paper wrap.

The Go To: (staples)

Sautéed broccoli and cauliflower. Cooked in ghee or sunflower oil with a generous dash of Indian spices. Add eggs or nutritional yeast for protein. Fill your plate and enjoy!

Indian spice mix: turmeric, ginger, fennel, cumin, coriander, fenugreek, black pepper and chili pepper. Garlic is great for Kapha dosha. (See appendix B for "Agni" spice blend)

Snacks: Reduce snacking. An apple, carrots, celery and herbal tea are best.

Sip: tea: ½ tsp ginger with ½ tsp cinnamon and a pinch of clove. Seep in hot water for 10 minutes. Can add honey to warm water (tea) for taste. Digestive tea: equal parts ginger, fennel, cumin and coriander. Seep ½ tsp in hot water for 5 minutes. (see appendix for blend). Drink mostly warm water. No juices or sodas. Sip peppermint, dandelion and nettle tea per preference.

In Your Fridge: Pre-cut and washed veggies (onions, tomatoes, kale, Brussels sprouts, arugula, broccoli, cauliflower, pepper and garlic), pre-cooked quinoa and millet,pre-soaked black beans, chickpeas and lentils. Pre-washed berries, cranberries,cherries, apples and other bitter and astringent fruits. Organic eggs, pre-baked organic chicken and freshwater fish.

In your pantry: sunflower oil, pumpkin seeds, cinnamon, spices, barley/millet/buckwheat (warm breakfast cereal) and ghee.

> *"Family Recipe: 3 cups of forgiveness, 1 gallon of friendship, 2 pinches of hope, a spoonful of laughter, oodles of love... mix, blend, repeat. Serve to everyone."*
>
> **—Anonymous**

Specific Foods to Favor and Avoid Per Dosha

Vata Pacifying Diet—Favor warm over cold, moist over dry, and grounding over light.

Eat: cooked apples, applesauce, apricots, bananas, berries, cantaloupe, cherries, coconut, dates, figs, grapes, kiwi, lemon, lime mangoes, melon, oranges, papaya, peaches, plums, avocado, beets, carrots, garlic, green beans, leeks, mustard greens, olives, peas, pumpkin, squash, sweet potatoes, zucchini, oats, pancakes, quinoa, wheat, lentils, miso, mung beans. soy, tofu, buttermilk, ghee, almonds, cashews, pine nuts, walnuts, beef, chicken, duck, eggs, salmon, sardines, shrimp, tuna, and turkey. Use avocado oil, ghee, olive oil, and sesame oil when preparing dishes. Spices: ginger, cumin, turmeric, cinnamon, black pepper, ajwan, hing, nutmeg, salt, thyme, and vanilla are best! Sweeten items with: date sugar, honey, jaguars, maple syrup, and molasses.

Avoid: Raw apples, green bananas, cranberries, persimmons, pomegranates, dried fruits, artichokes, bell peppers, bitter melon, broccoli (raw especially), Brussels sprouts, cabbage, cauliflower (raw especially), celery, corn, dandelion greens, kale, lettuce, raw onion, hot peppers, raw spinach, tomatoes, barley, buckwheat, couscous, millet, rice cakes, black beans, garbanzo beans, navy beans, white beans. frozen yogurt, powdered milk, popcorn, lamb, pork, rabbit, and venison. Avoid canola oil,corn oil, and soy oil when preparing dishes.

Pitta Pacifying Diet—Favor cooling over heating, dry or oily, and satiating over light.

Eat: apples, apricots, berries, cherries, coconut, dates, grapes, mangoes, melons, sweet oranges (not sour), pears, sweet pineapple (not sour), prunes, raisins, strawberry, watermelon, avocado, artichoke, asparagus, beets, bitter melon, cabbage, carrots, sprouts, cilantro, collard greens, dandelion greens, green beans, kale, leafy greens, lettuce, mushrooms, okra, peas, parsnips, spaghetti squash, summer squash, sweet potatoes, wheatgrass, zucchini, barley, couscous, granola, oats, pancakes, basmati rice, wild rice, wheat, black beans, kidney beans, lentils, soy, tempeh, tofu, white beans, ghee, goats milk, coconut, unsalted popcorn, pumpkin seeds, white meat chicken, egg whites, freshwater fish, shrimp, white meat turkey, and venison. Use coconut oil, ghee, and olive oil when preparing dishes. Spices: basil, cardamom, cumin, fennel, ginger, mint, turmeric, vanilla, and wintergreen are best! Sweeten items with: barley malt, date sugar, rice syrup, and stevia.

Avoid: Sour apples, sour berries/cherries/oranges/pineapple/plums, burdock root, corn, radish, garlic, chilies, horseradish, mustard greens, raw onions, olives, capers, hot peppers, tomatoes, turnips, buckwheat, corn, millet, brown rie, rye, miso, soy sauce, sour cream, butter, yogurt, chia seeds, peanuts, sesame seeds, tahini, walnuts, beef, dark chicken, egg yolks, salmon, pork, sardines, seafoods, tuna, and dark meat turkey. Avoid corn oil and sesame oil when preparing dishes.

Kapha Pacifying Diet—Favor warming over cooling, dry over moist, and light over heavy.

Eat: apples, berries, cranberries, cherries, lemons, limes, mango, peaches, pears, persimmons, pomegranates, prunes, raspberries, strawberries, artichokes, asparagus, beet greens, bell peppers, bitter melon, broccoli, Brussels sprouts, burdock root, cauliflower, celery, chilies, cilantro, amaranth, barley, buckwheat, couscous, millet, oat bran, quinoa, rice cakes, sprouted wheat bread (ezekiel), black beans, black-eye peas, chickpeas, lentils, navy beans, split peas, tempeh, tofu, white beans, ghee, skim goat's milk, chia seeds, flax seeds, pumpkin seeds, sunflower seeds, white meat chicken, egg whites, shrimp, rabbit, and white meat turkey. Use almond oil, flax seed oil, ghee, and sunflower oil when preparing dishes. Spices: Ajwan, anise, basil, bay leaf, black pepper, cardamom, cayenne, cinnamon, cumin, fennel, fenugreek, garlic, ginger, nutmeg, peppermint, turmeric, and wintergreen are best! Sweeten with: honey and raw fruit juices.

Avoid: bananas, cantaloupe, coconut, dates, figs, green grapes, grapefruit, melons, oranges, pineapple, plums, watermelon, avocado, cucumber, pumpkin, squash, sweet potatoes, zucchini, cooked oats, pancakes, pasta, rice, wheat, bread, kidney beans, miso, soy products, cold tofu, soy sauce, butter, cheese, milk, cream, yogurt, brazil nuts, cashews, macadamia nuts, pistachios, sesame seeds, tahini, walnuts, beef, dark meat chicken/turkey, lamb, pork, sardines, tuna, salmon, and saltwater fish (in excess). Avoid using too much oil when preparing dishes.

"People who love what they eat are the best people."

—Julia Child

Healthy Recipes

Curated from various online blogs, painters, health sites and cookbooks.

Next to each recipe you will see the letters V, P and K. As you have probably gathered this will stand for Vata, Pitta and Kapha. If you see a (+) sign next to the letter that means it will increase that Dosha. If you see a (-) sign that means it will decrease that Dosha. If you see a (=) sign that means it will neither increase nor decrease the Dosha. You'll see that the majority of the recipes are suitable for all three Doshas.

If you have an imbalance you want to choose the recipes that decrease the aggravating Dosha. For example if I have heartburn, loose stools, acne and have been impatient, I have a Pitta imbalance. I want to choose recipes that have the symbol (P-). All of these recipes contain whole food, fresh ingredients and can be enjoyed by everyone in moderation so long as there is no serious imbalance or pre-existing condition.

YUMMIES!

(suitable for breakfasts, snacks and desserts)

Date Milk Shake (K+, V-, P-)

Ingredients:

- A pinch of cinnamon
- 4-5 whole dates
- 1 cup almond milk.

Directions: Put almond milk, cinnamon and dates in automatic blender. Blend until dates are ground fine.

Rice Pudding (K+, V-, P-)

Ingredients:

- 1 cup water
- ½ cup basmati rice
- 4 cups almond milk
- 1 tsp. chopped dates
- 2 tsp. cashews or pistachios
- 3 small pieces green cardamom crushed
- 1 tsp. sugar (or to taste

Directions: Soak rice in water for 2 hours. Boil almond milk. Add rice and all other ingredients. Boil slowly for 30 minutes or more until the mixture reaches a slightly thick consistency, but you can stir it easily. It will thicken a little more when you let it cool.

Carrot and Oat Balls (suitable for all 3 Doshas!)

Ingredients:

- » 1 cup steel cut oats
- » 1.5 cups carrots
- » 1 cup pitted dates
- » 1/3 cup ground flaxseed
- » 1 tsp golden milk
- » powder
- » 1 tbs organic honey

Directions: Combine ingredients in food processor for about 30 seconds to create a paste. Pour into a mixing bowl and add 1 cup dry organic oats. Roll the dough into big generous size balls.Store in the refrigerator and grab a few for breakfast or keep them in a mini fridge at work and grab one for an afternoon snack.

Banana Oat Breakfast Balls (K+, V-, P=)

Ingredients:

- » 4 large, very ripe bananas
- » 4 cups large flake oats (old-fashioned oats), gluten-free if necessary
- » ½ cup unsweetened shredded coconut
- » ½ cup ground hazelnuts or almonds or more coconut—optional
- » ½ cup mini chocolate chips
- » 1 teaspoon baking powder

- 2 teaspoons vanilla
- 2 teaspoons cinnamon

Directions: Preheat the oven to 350°F. Line a baking sheet with parchment paper, or lightly grease it. Mash the bananas in a large bowl with a potato masher or a fork. Combine all ingredients and blend (a food processor works marvels). Roll dough into bite size balls, place them 1.5 inches apart on a lubricated baking pan. Bake for 10-12 minutes. This recipe is flexible. Use wiggle room to play around and create!

Golden Milk Date Balls (K+, V-, P-)

Ingredients:

- 1 cup almonds
- 1 cup pitted dates
- ½ cup unsweetened
- coconut
- ½ cup organic cacao
- 1 tbs golden milk powder
- (turmeric/ginger/cinnamon/cardamom/nutmeg)

Directions: Combine ingredients in a food processor and blend for about 30 seconds. You may need to add 1 tbs of organic honey if your paste isn't very sticky. Roll the dough into bite size balls and enjoy! (These directions create 12-16 balls)

Golden Milk (suitable for all 3 Doshas)

(Calms nervous system, reduced inflammation and aids in restful sleep. Great for all doshas and kids.) Heat one cup of almond/cashew/soy/rice or hemp milk with ½ tsp ginger powder, ½ tsp turmeric powder and a dash of cinnamon, nutmeg and cardamom. Serve warm. (see appendix for pre-made blend)

Ojas Milk (K+, P-, V-)

(Calms nervous system and increases immunity. Great for Vata Dosha and kids.) One cup of warm almond/cashew/soy/rice or hemp milk with 4 pitted dates and four almonds. Add ¼ tsp of each: cinnamon, ginger, cardamom and nutmeg powders, blend in a blender and enjoy!

SUSTENANCE:

Curry Chickpea Stew (K-,P+, V-)

Ingredients:

- 1 tsp olive oil
- 1 white onion, diced
- 3 cloves garlic, minced
- 1 tbsp fresh ginger
- 1 tsp curry powder
- 1 tsp turmeric
- 2 tbsp Thai curry paste (lemongrass and chili/ buy at asian or local grocery store)
- 4 carrots, peeled and chopped

» 1.5 lb. potato, chopped into roughly 1" pieces (russet, red, baby or even sweet potato is ok)
» ½ crown cauliflower, chopped
» 1 cup coconut milk
» 2 cup vegetable stock
» 1.5 cups green peas
» 1 x 28 oz. can chickpeas (approx. 3 cups cooked chickpeas)

Directions: In a saucepan, sauté the onion and garlic in the olive oil for a few minutes. Add the garlic, ginger, spices and curry paste and continue stirring. Add all the veggies and continue cooking and stirring for about 5 minutes. Add the stock and coconut and simmer over low heat for approximately 20-30 minutes or until the potato is cooked through. Stir in the peas and chickpeas, turn off the heat and let sit for another 5 minutes. Serve.

Barley and Kale Moroccan Salad (K-, P=, V+)

Ingredients:

» 1 cup barley uncooked
» 5 cups kale, pre-stemmed and cut into small pieces
» 1 cup parsley, finely chopped
» 1 red pepper, diced
» ½ cup raisins
» ½ cup raw pistachio kernels, unsalted
» For the Dressing:

- 4 cloves garlic
- 3 tbsp fresh lemon juice
- 2 tbsp apple cider vinegar
- 1 tsp cumin
- 1 tsp turmeric
- ½ tsp paprika
- 3 tbsp olive oil
- 1 tsp maple syrup
- 1 tbsp water
- salt and pepper to taste

Directions: Cook the barley according to instructions.Add the kale, parsley and red pepper to a large bowl and mix well. Add the dressing ingredients to a blender or food processor, or use an immersion blender and mix until smooth. Pour over the kale mixture, stirring until the kale is well coated. Once the barley is cooked, drain any excess water and add to the rest of the ingredients. Fold in the raisins and pistachios. Enjoy!

Red Curry Rice and Lentil Stew (K-, P+, V-)

Ingredients:

- 1 onion, diced
- 4 cloves garlic, minced
- 1 tbsp fresh ginger, minced
- 3 tbsp of red curry paste
- 4 carrots, peeled and chopped

- 1 head of cauliflower, cut into florets
- 1 tbsp soy sauce or tamarin
- ½ cup jasmine rice
- ½ cup uncooked red lentils
- 1⅓ cup vegetable stock
- 1 (28 oz.) can diced tomatoes, with their juices
- 1 tsp brown sugar
- salt and pepper, to taste

Directions: In a large sauce pan, cook the garlic, onion and ginger over medium heat for minutes, stirring.Add the carrots, cauliflower and red curry paste. Stir and cook for a few more minutes.Add the rest of the ingredients, stir, cover and lightly simmer for 20 minutes. Remove the lid and let simmer for another 5-10 minutes until everything is cooked and most of the liquid is absorbed.

Bell Pepper Chickpea Salad with Tahini Dressing (K-, P=, V+)

Ingredients:

- 1 tbsp lemon
- 3 tbsp extra-virgin olive oil
- 3 tbsp tahini
- 2 tbsp white wine vinegar
- 3 cloves garlic, minced
- 1 tsp smoked paprika
- ½ tsp salt
- ½ tsp pepper

- 1 yellow pepper, diced
- 1 red pepper, diced
- 1 green pepper, diced
- 2 can chickpeas, drained and well-rinsed
- 1 cucumber, peeled and diced
- 2 cups lightly packed parsley, finely chopped
- ½ cup raisins

Directions: Place all ingredients in a large bowl and mix well. Store any leftovers in the fridge for up to 3 days.

Lemongrass and Garlic Chickpea Salad (K-, P=, V+)

Ingredients:

- ¼ cup fresh rosemary, finely chopped
- 5 cloves garlic, minced
- 1 cup fresh parsley finely chopped
- 2 tbsp olive oil
- 3 tbsp fresh lemon juice
- 2 x 19 oz can chickpeas, drained and well rinsed
- ½ tsp sea salt
- ½ tsp fresh ground black peppercorns

Directions: Add everything to a bowl and mix well.

Spicy Creamy Tomato Soup (K-, P+, V-)

Ingredients:

- » ¾ cup unsweetened almond milk
- » ½ cup raw cashews, soaked at least 2 hours
- » 1 tbsp olive oil
- » 1 onion, diced
- » 6 cloves garlic, minced
- » 3 tbsp fresh dill, finely chopped
- » ½ tsp crushed chili flakes (optional)
- » ½ tsp black pepper, or to taste
- » ½ tsp salt, or to taste
- » 1—28 oz can diced tomato
- » 1 cup vegetable stock

Directions: Place the almond milk and cashews in a blender and process until completely smooth.In a soup pot, sauté the onions and garlic in the olive oil for about 5 minutes. Add the rest of the ingredients, including the cashew mixture, stir well and continue cooking for 10 minutes. Use an immersion blender or transfer the soup to a blender and blend until smooth. Serve topped with lots of fresh dill and chopped fresh tomato.

Spicy Vegan Chili (K-,P+, V-)

Ingredients:

- » 2 tbsp extra virgin olive oil
- » 1 white onion, diced
- » 5 cloves garlic, diced
- » 3 tbsp chili powder
- » 2 bay leaves
- » 1 6 oz. can tomato paste
- » 5 carrots, chopped
- » 1 jalepeno, seeded and diced
- » 1 red pepper, diced
- » 1 green pepper, diced
- » 1 yellow pepper, diced
- » 1 19 oz. can black beans, drained and rinsed
- » 1 19 oz. can fava beans, drained and rinsed
- » 1 19 oz. can kidney beans, drained and rinsed
- » 1 tsp sea salt
- » 1 tsp black pepper
- » 1 vegetable bouillon cube
- » 1—1½ cup water (start with 1 cup and add a little extra if it's too thick)
- » 1 crown of cauliflower, grated (approx. 3 cups)

Directions: Cook the onion and garlic in the olive oil for 5 minutes, stirring. Add the chili powder, bay leaves and tomato paste and cook for a few more minutes. Add in all the vegetables, except for the cauliflower. Add the water and bouillon cube, cover and simmer about 10 minutes. Add the grated cauliflower and continue to cook until all the vegetables are soft and the chili is nice and thick. (Approx. 10-20 minutes). Remove the bay leaves and serve. Makes 4 huge servings or 6-8 smaller portions.

Summer Cream of Squash (V-, P-, K+)

Ingredients for 4 people:

» 2 big organic squashes or 3 medium ones (any summer squash will do—I used the combination on the picture above)

» one small sweet onion

» 4 garlic cloves

» 1 teaspoon white sesame seeds

» ½ teaspoon of Agni spice blend

» 1 Rapunzel veggie bouillon cube (or other organic, non GMO bouillon cube)

» 2 cups of water

» 2 tablespoons organic sour cream or plain greek yogurt (unsweetened)

» Fresh mint and basil (or lemon balm)

Directions: Cut the previously washed squashes and onion into medium size cubes (2 inches wide or so). Peel the garlic, and cut in half each clove. In a pot or pressure cooker, add all cut veggies along with the bouillon cube, the sesame seed, the spice blend and the water. If using a pressure cooker, once the steam comes out, cook for 10 minutes. If using a conventional pot, cook covered until squashes are tender, but not overly cooked. Mix all the ingredients in a blender, adding the sour cream and fresh basil and mint (you may use a few leaves of each herb up to ¼ cup minced herb mix, depending on taste). Voilà! Enjoy warm, room temperature or cold.

Sunflower Kale Salad (V+, P-, K-)

Ingredients, for 8 people:

» 2 bunches kale

» ¼ C Seasame oil

» 2/3 C Sunflower seeds, roasted

» 3 TBS Tamari or Braggs aminio acid

* For Pitta use ghee or coconut oil

**Kale can be substituted for collard greens

Directions: Remove stems from kale, wash and chop the leaves. Roast sunflower seeds in a warm, dry pan until lightly browned. Put aside. Warm oil in a saucepan, add in kale. Sauté until kale is coated with oil. Add sunflower seeds and tamari. Stir to coat. Serve warm!

Coconut Quinoa Rice and Vegetables (V-, P-, K-)

Ingredients:

» 5 cups mixed vegetables chopped: carrots and broccoli (use any summer vegetable)

» ½ tablespoon ginger chopped

- ½ cup white basmati rice
- ½ cup quinoa
- 1 cup coconut milk
- 1 ½ cups water
- ¼ cup shredded unsweetened coconut
- Salt to taste

Directions: Cook the rice, quinoa, ginger, and vegetables in the coconut milk/water mixture (stovetop or rice cooker) until cooked. In a skillet, dry roast the shredded coconut over low heat until golden brown and fragrant. Add the coconut and salt and gently stir into the coconut/rice/quinoa mixture. Serve warm with cilantro and mint chutney and/or roasted papads (Indian lentil wafers); Also can be served as an accompaniment for fish or meat dishes.

Cucumber, Watermelon & Mint Salad (V+, P-, K+)

Ingredients:

- 2 cups cubed cucumber (English or Persian)
- 2 cups cubed watermelon (de-seeded)
- Juice of 2 limes
- 3-4 tablespoons chopped fresh mint
- Salt to taste

Directions: Combine above ingredients in a bowl. Serve slightly cool. Optional: Sprinkle crumbled goat or feta cheese just before serving. Chef's note: If making salad ahead of time, do not add lime juice and salt until just before serving

"The more you let Ayurveda and Yoga become the basis for your living, the easier life becomes."

—Mayra Lewin

SIMPLE AYURVEDIC RECIPES FOR EVERYONE

From Simple Ayurvedic Recipes by Myra Lewin

Quinoa with Apples

1 ½ cups quinoa, 4 cups water, 1 tbsp ghee, ½ tsp mineral salt, 1 3 inch cinnamon stick, 3/4 tsp coriander powder, 1-2 cup chopped apples... combine and bring to boil, cover lid, reduce to simmer for 10-15 minutes.

Dhal Soup

1-2 tbsp ghee, 1-2 tsp grated ginger, 1 tsp grated turmeric, 1 ½ tsp cumin seeds, ¼ tsp asafetida, 1 tsp mineral salt, 1 cup split mung beans, 4 cups water...heat ghee in sauce pan, add spices, cook until aroma comes up, add beans, add water, stir and bring to boil. Reduce to simmer and cover with a lid for 25 mins.

Garbanzo Beans with Coconut

1 cup garbanzo beans, 1 tbs sesame oil, ¼ tsp asafetida, ½ tsp mineral salt, 1 pinch ginger powder, 2 tsp powdered coriander, ½ ts, ground cinnamon, ½ tsp ground black pepper, water, ½ cup coconut milk...combine all ingredients together (except coconut milk) in a pot. Add water to cover the beans 1/3 inch and stir.

Bring to a boil, reduce to simmer, and cover with a lid for 35-45 mins. Add coconut milk after garbanzo beans are cooked.

Carrot Ginger Soup

3 cups chopped carrot, 1 tbsp ghee, 2 tsp fresh grated ginger (powder is ok), ¼ cup whole organic milk (optional) or almond milk, ½ cup cilantro, ½ tsp black pepper, water...cut carrots and add water to 3/4 the level of them in the pot. Add ghee. Simmer until carrots are soft. Cool a little. Place carrots in liquid in blender and add milk and cilantro. Blend until smooth or leave a few chunks of carrots. Stir in black pepper at the end.

Pumpkin Soup

2 tbsp ghee, 2 tsp ginger, 1 tsp turmeric, ½ tsp mineral salt, 1 tsp black pepper, 1 tsp cumin seeds, ½ tsp powdered cardamom, 3 cups chopped pumpkin, water...heat ghee on medium heat and add spices, cook until the spices' aroma comes up. Add pumpkin and stir to coat with ghee and spices. Add water to 1/3 the level of pumpkin and stir, and cover with a lid. Reduce the heat and simmer 10-15 mins or until pumpkin is soft. Blend all or part of the pumpkin in the blender.

Quinoa Balls

1 cup cooked split Mung beans, 1 cup cooked quinoa, ghee, sesame oil or coconut oil...form split mung into balls, coat with quinoa. Warm in an oiled pan with ghee, sesame or coconut oil. Eat in a wrap with an avocado.

CHAPTER SEVENTEEN

Home Remedies

"The art of medicine is amusing the patient while nature cures the disease."

—Voltaire

HOME REMEDIES FOR Common Imbalances: These home remedies are meant to be used in concert with whatever medical plan you subscribe to. This information is not intended to substitute for medical advice. While Ayurveda is amazing at preventing imbalances and creating harmony within the mind-body, some imbalances are beyond the scope of unsupervised self-healing. Use your logic, and intuition. Seek a practitioner for guidance.

What is Neti Pot? A neti pot is a small tea-like device designed to rinse your nasal passage from allergens, reside, and debris. You can purchase one at your local drugstore or online. To use a neti pot, fill the container with slightly warm temperature water and add ½ teaspoon of salt to the pot. Tilt your head sideways over the sink and pour the contents of the container through your upper nostril. The liquid will exit through the lower nostril. Breathe through the mouth. Then repeat on the other side. Once your finished, bend over the bathtub or go outside and blow the excess fluid out of both nostrils by taking thirty vibrant exhalations through the nose. I find that using a neti pot in the morning is best. This practice will help with sinus issues, congestion, allergies, and colds.

» **Acne:** Avoid sugar, dairy, and spicy foods. Use Radiant Me Complexion Mask by wellBlends, and dab tea tree oil onto effected spots. Be sure to drink plenty of water. Generally, you'll want to follow a Pitta pacifying diet because acne is heat and inflammation. If you have cystic acne, you'll want to want to be specific about avoid all dairy foods. This includes: milk, cheese, yogurt, sour cream, ice cream, and heavy cream in coffee. The skin can also become angry if we're angry. Reflect inward and see if you are dealing with unexpressed anger. Finally, the skin can be a representation of how we see ourselves. Check in with yourself and acknowledge and perhaps shift the way you're viewing yourself. Your affirmation can be, "I am beautiful inside and out." Acne is associated with the seventh chakra.

» **Anxiety:** Vata pacifying diet, golden milk, chamomile tea, meditation, alternate nostril breathing, and herbs such as abhwagandha. Anxiety is a Vata type imbalance that is often caused by too much travel, instability, change, over crowded schedules, and fear. See if you can simplify your schedule, ground by sitting outside on the earth, or walking with bare feet, and breath. Anxiety is usually connected to reminiscing about the past, or projecting into the future.

Becoming present quells anxiety. Breathing is a great passage to the present moment. You can inhale for four counts. Pause, and hold your breath for four counts, and exhale for four counts. Try to breathe through the nose. Do this at least three times and you'll feel the waves of ease.

» **Arthritis:** Golden milk, Epsom salt baths, and herbs such as triphala and goggulu. Arthritis is caused by inflammation and toxicity in the joints. Be specific about avoiding processed foods because the chemicals and additives cause inflammation and toxicity. Drink plenty of warm water with lemon to help flush out toxins.

» **Asthma:** Drink Half a cup of ginger tea mixed with 2-3 crushed garlic cloves to pacify an attack. Drink Golden milk, or licorice tea, and follow a generally Kapha pacifying diet. Asthma is associated with the heart chakra.

» **Bloating:** ginger/cumin/coriander/fennel tea (Detox & Replenish Tea by wellBlends), a Vata pacifying diet, making sure you eat fruit alone as a snack (never with other items), avoid incompatible foods, and eat slowly. Eating in a hurry or while we're emotional disturbed impairs digestion and can lead to bloating. Be sure to slow down and clear your mind before you eat. Bloating is associated with the third chakra.

» **(High) Blood Pressure:** Add a teaspoon of coriander and a pinch of cardamom to one cup of freshly squeezed peach juice. Drink this 2-3 times a day. Take 2 tablespoons of ground flaxseed daily. Practice yoga because it blends relaxation with exercise. Both of these aims will help bring your blood pressure down.

» **Back Pain:** Vata pacifying diet, warm oil massage, Epsom salt bath, reclined spinal twists, supported bridge pose, and golden milk. Back pain is often associated with the first chakra. Are you feeling financially and physically safe, secure, and provided for? Grounding and practicing affirmations around abundance and stability are helpful. Example: Sit on the earth, take three deep breaths, feel the earth hold and support you. Say to yourself, "I am safe and supported. My life is full and abundant. Everything I need is here or coming to me now."

» **Candida:** Drink ginger tea, or wellBlends detox & replenish tea, sip hot water throughout the day, and avoid cold and heavy foods. Eliminate sugar and refined carbohydrates. Put 6 drops of organic oil of oregano under your tongue. Oil of oregano is anti-fungal. You can try herbs such as grape seed extract, bhrami, and aloe vera,

» **Cough:** Drink honey tea, ginger tea, and gargle salt water.

» **Cold:** Chew on ginger, use a Neti pot, and drink hot water regularly.

» **Congestion:** Use a Neti pot, and Nasya oil (Clarity oil by wellBlends), and follow a Kapha pacifying diet to reduce mucus and phlegm.

» **Cold Sores:** Apply ice, dab on lemon juice 2-3 times a day, and take salt on a wet finger and apply it to the sore by pressing for 30 seconds. Irritation may occur, but it will help it heal.

» **Constipation:** Follow a generally Vata pacifying diet, take 2 tablespoons of aloe vera gel concentrate before bed, and drink golden milk. If it is severe, add 1 tablespoon of ghee to hot water and drink it first thing in the morning, or drink senna leaf tea. Triphala is helpful as well. Constipation is associated with the first chakra. Often times constipation is caused by not giving ourselves time to have a movement. Slow down in the morning. Breathe and relax. Also, constipation is common while traveling. Again, we're out of our routine and in a new environment. When traveling as well, give yourself time and space to relax in the morning so your body feels safe to release.

» **Diabetes:** Follow a generally Kapha pacifying diet. Drink Golden Milk and use it in cooking. To regulate blood sugar; take ½ a teaspoon of ground bay leaf and ½ a teaspoon of turmeric, mixed with one tablespoon of aloe vera gel concentrate.

» **Dry skin:** Give yourself daily oil massages, follow a generally Vata pacifying diet, and drink plenty of warm water.

» **Dandruff:** Mix a small amount of camphor essential oil with coconut oil and massage it into your hair before bed.

» **Diarrhea:** Drink ginger tea with cumin added to it once a day, eat unripped bananas with a large pinch of nutmeg, and avoid all cold food/drink items.Diarrhea is associated with the first chakra.

» **Eczema:** Apply aloe vera gel directly from the plant, massage skin with coconut oil, and try dabbing local organic honey onto the affected area. Follow a generally Vata-Pitta pacifying diet, meaning eat warm grounding foods that are not spicy or acidic. Skin issues are associated with the seventh chakra.

» **Fever:** Gargle salt water, use Neti pot, and sip hot water every 20 minutes throughout the day. Eat only ver light foods like miso soup, or broth.

» **Gas:** Drink ginger/cumin/coriander/fennel tea (Detox & Replenish Tea), avoid cold fluids, and never eat fruit after a meal. Follow Vata pacifying diet and lifestyle guidelines. Gas is too much ether and air (Vata) in the body.

» **Gerd:** Limit salads, fatty foods, fried foods, carbonated drinks, and Pitta irritating foods like garlic, onions, and vinegar. Eat food slowly, and drink tea made with boiled water and cumin seeds. Gerd is associated with the throat chakra.

» **Heartburn:** Drink Detox & Replenish Tea, Don't snack if you're not hungry, follow a generally Pitta pacifying diet, and drink coconut water or aloe vera juice. Heartburn is associated with the fourth chakra.

» **Hair Loss:** Take herbs such as amalaki, bhringaraj, or "Healthy Hair" by Banyan Botanicals. Follow a generally Pitta pacifying lifestyle, meditate, and give yourself coconut oil massages. People with Pitta constitutions are more prone to premature graying and hair loss.

» **Hot Flashes:** Avoid Pitta irritating foods, take 2 tablespoons of aloe vera gel concentrate before bed, and try herbs such as shatavari and amalaki.

» **Headache:** Hydrate, do a restorative yoga practice, and try diffusing peppermint essential oil into the air, or dab the oil on your wrists. Headaches are associated with the third eye chakra, or the seat of your intuition. The headache is a signal that something needs your attention. Check in to see what your intuition is trying to tell you: do you need to shift environments, re-evaluate your job or a relationships? Also, headaches can be associated with dehydration and sensitivity to light. Drink plenty of water and avoid excess light exposure. Seek shade on sunny days. Headaches are associated with the sixth chakra.

» **Inflammation:** Avoid sugar, dairy, processed grains, fried foods, and red meat. Drink Golden Milk, and add frankincense oil to your baths

» **Insomnia:** Set regular wake and sleep cycles. Try to go to bed and wake up at the same time each day. Unplug 30-60minutes before bed. Drink Golden milk before bed. Practice Yoga Nidra, guided sleep meditation (can use the Insight Timer app). Supplements alone will not cure insomnia. You'll need to shift your lifestyle, but you can try ashwagandha, melatonin, and magnesium to support sleep. Insomnia is a Vata imbalance. Make sure you simplify your schedule, calm your mind and nervous system with pranayama, and ground in nature each day.

» **Irregular Periods:** Follow a Vata pacifying diet, adopt regular routines that integrate balanced proportions of rest and activity, try Women's Support herbal compound by Banyan Botanicals. Practice alternate nostril breathing for 2-5 minutes morning and night to help balance your hormones. Pay attention to your second chakra. Practice hip openers and Yin yoga. Our menstrual cycle is typically a print out of all our cycles and rhythms. If our period cycle is not consistent it often means we need more consistency in our lives. A morning and evening routine of self-care that is practiced religiously for 30-60 days should help restore a more stable rhythm. Irregular periods are associated with the second chakra. "Women's Support" by Banyan Botanicals may prove beneficial for you.

» **Kidney Stones:** Drink 64 ounces of water, Have two 5-ounce glasses of lemon juice on an empty stomach in the morning, drink 2-8 ounces of wheat grass juice, or try 5 ounces of extra-virgin olive oil first thing in the morning and late in the afternoon. This may reduce pain and discomfort.

» **(Low) Blood Pressure:** Eat small portions of food more frequently, consume an adequate amount of salt, and drink 2-3 liters of water daily.

» **Liver Issues:** Meditate to address anger and resentment, take cooling herbs like neem and aloe vera, and eat lots of leafy greens. Leafy greens are bitter, so they help to cool and detoxify the liver. The liver is associated with anger and resentment. Reflect inward and see if these hot emotions need an outlet such as music, exercise, or expression through conversation or journaling. As Dr.Lad said, the underlining cause of diseases are repressed emotions. Give yourself a safe outlet.

» **Menstrual Cramps:** Drink Golden Milk, massage with sesame oil, apply heat, and take a bath with lavender. Pay attention to second chakra, and make sure you're incorporating plenty of rest and downtime (Yin) into your lifestyle. Our cycle is a print out of how much Yin (being, receiving, restoring) verses Yang (doing, giving, activity) we have in our lives. Ideally, we want the amount of Yin and Yang/ Doing and Being to be about even. If the scales are tipped too far in one direction, our period will let us know. In todays modern world, most of us are too Yang. We're over active and this burns up our Yin fluids. If your cramps are awful, try adding in more Yin yoga and self-care and see what happens. Menstrual cramps are associated with the second chakra.

» **Migraines:** Follow a Vata-Pitta pacifying diet (grounding foods that are not spicy.) Diffuse peppermint and lavender oils into the air, hydrate, and do a slow yoga practice. Pay attention to your third eye charkra, and ask your intuition, "What are you here to teach me?"

» **Osteoporosis:** Follow a Vata pacifying diet, take magnesium with calcium, try ashwagandha, eat sesame seeds with molasses, lift very light weights, and practice Hatha yoga. Osteoporosis is associated with the seventh chakra. (All skin, nervous system, and skeletal issues are seventh chakra.)

» **Ovarian Cysts:** Drink Golden Milk, try herbs like triphala and guggul, and apply castor oil packs before bed. Ovarian cysts, and anything pertaining to our reproductive organs are associated with second chakra.

» **Reflux:** Follow a Pitta pacifying diet, cook with cilantro/ coriander/mint, eat slowly, and avoid ice. Acid reflux is a blend of third and fourth chakra.

» **Ringing in the ears (Tinnitus):** Apply 10 drops of sesame oil in each ear daily. Follow a Vata pacifying diet and lifestyle, and avoid the cold and wind. Tinnitus is associated with the third eye chakra.

- » **Sinus Infection:** Use a Neti pot, use Nasya (Clarity oil by wellBlends), drink plenty of water, and apply a warm compress to your face. Sinus infections and anything related to ears, nose, and eyes are associated with the sixth chakra.
- » **Sore Throat:** Gargle salt water, use a Neti pot, and chew on ginger.
- » **Thyroid issues:** Meditate to restore the adrenal glands (the counterpart to the thyroid), avoid sugar, practice shoulder stand (yoga pose), and pay attention to your throat chakra. Are you speaking your truth and feeling understood?
- » **Urinary Tract Infection:** Follow a generally Pitta pacifying diet; avoid alcohol, spicy, and sour foods. Drink plenty of water, practice bridge pose, bow pose, and cobra pose to stimulate kidney functions, and make sure you always urinate after having sex.
- » **Ulcer:** Follow a Pitta pacifying diet, drink licorice tea, and take 1 tablespoon of aloe vera gel concentrate. Practice alternate nostril breathing, and daily meditation. Make sure you're taking time to refresh and play. Ulcers are often the result of overworking. Ulcers are associated with the third chakra.
- » **Vomiting:** Drink ginger tea, hydrate, and chew on one or two cardamom seeds.
- » **Yeast Infection:** Avoid alcohol, dairy, coffee, sugar, and processed grains. Try taking a good pro-biotic. Preferably one that is 100 billion microbes. And you can mix 6 drops of oregano oil with 1 teaspoon of coconut oil and apply it to vaginal wall daily. Yeast infections are related to second chakra.

Closing Regards...

I hope the pages of this book have come alive for you. I know Yoga is a trusted companion in your life. It is my hope that Ayurveda has effectuality made its mark on your life, and has become a friend as well. The merging of Ayurveda and Yoga together offer a tremendous level of support that we cannot get from one or the other on their own. May these two sciences blend seamlessly into your life. May their support be readily available and frequently accessed as you see fit. Ayurveda is the Science of Life, and as we know, life is constantly changing and evolving. As you shift through the many colorful seasons, situations, and stages of life, keep your Ayurveda and Yoga practices with you. Should you fall out of balance, return to the basics. Using your life as medicine is as much of an art as it is a science. With all art, there will always be freedom, individuality, and beauty. These faculties are yours—now and always.

> *"Create the highest grandest vision for your life. Then let every step move you in that direction."*
>
> **—Oprah Winfrey**

ABOUT YOUR AUTHOR

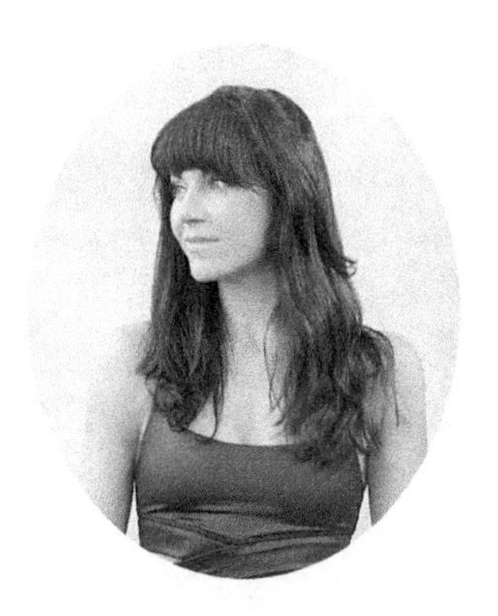

KRISTEN SCHNEIDER IS an international yoga teacher, board certified Ayurveda Practitioner, and three time author. She studied yoga in China and India, and earned her 500RYT in Rishikesh, India. She studied Ayurveda at the Kripalu School of Ayurveda, The Ayurveda Institute, and The Chakrapani Research Clinic in Jaipur, India. She is the creator of wellBlends, an organic line of Ayurvedic products for self-care, and owns Ayurveda Orlando—a holistic clinic in Orlando, Florida. Kristen currently lives in Tampa, Florida. Her newest book, Love Fearlessly: The Soulmate Within is now available.

social: @kristenschneider

contact@wellblends.com

www.wellblends.com

APPENDIX A.

Resources for Products and Inspiration & Reccomended Reading...

Wellblends, Organic Ayurvedic Products for Self-Care: www.wellblends.com

Summary of Products (uses & benefits)

Golden Milk: Helps reduce inflammation, promotes proper sleep and optimal digestion. Ingredients: turmeric, ginger, cardamom, cinnamon and nutmeg. Put 1 tsp in hot almond milk and drink before bed. (You can also add a tsp to smoothies or to hot coffee with 1 tsp of coconut oil...this alleviates constipation too)

Detox and Replenish Tea: Relieves gas and bloating, increases absorption of nutrients and boosts digestive capacity. Ingredients: ginger, cumin, coriander and fennel. Put ½ tsp in 8oz of hot water and drink before meals.

Agni Spice: Makes whole foods taste great! Improves metabolism, digestion and absorption. Ingredients: ginger, turmeric, black pepper, coriander, cumin, cayenne and cinnamon. Use in/on stir-fry, beans, omelettes, tofu, chicken, fish and roasted veggies.

Clarity Oil: Clears sinuses, relieves allergies, quells anxiety and promotes focus. Ingredients: bhrami oil, lavender, eucalyptus and lemon organic oils. Use a q-tip to swab nose and ears (like you're cleaning your ears) morning and night.

Radiant Me Complexion Mask: Helps clear acne and blemishes, brings luster to skin and corrects discoloration of skin tone. Ingredients: neem, manjistha, triphala, turmeric and chickpea flour. Blends 1 tbs of powder with 1 tbs of water to create a paste. Cleanse face. Massage the paste into the skin and leave for 15 minutes. Rinse with warm water. Use 3-5x per week.

Herbs and Medicated Oils from:

www.banyanbotanicals.com

Resources for Meditation:

- Online meditations davidji.com and chopracentermeditation.com
- Smartphone Apps: Headspace and Insight Timer
- Wherever You Go There You Are by: Jon Kabat Zinn
- Meditate Your Weight by: Tiffany Cruikshank

Resources for Emotional Eating:

- Feeding the Hungry Heart
- and Breaking Free from Emotional Eating by: Geneen Roth
- What Are You Hungry For? by: Deepak Chopra

Resources for Recipes and Cookbooks

» The 25 Day Ayurveda Cleanse by: Kerry Harling
» Eat Feel Fresh by: Sahara Rose Ketabi
» Eat, Taste, Heal by: Thomas Yarema
» Make Your Own Rules Diet by: Tara Stiles
» Simple Ayurvedic Recipes by: Myra Lewin
» Ayurveda Cooking for Self Healing by: Usha Lad and Dr. Vasant Lad
» Aim True by: Kathryn Budig
» Online Sources: www.runningonrealfood.com and www.joyfulbelly.com

Resources for Nutrition:

» Ultra-Metabolism by: Mark Hyman
» The China Study by: T. Collin Campbell and Thomas M. Campbell
» In Defense of Food by: Michael Pollan
» How Not to Die by: Michael Greger M.D.

Inspiration:

» Return to Love by: Marianne Williamson
» Change Your Thoughts—Change Your Life by: Wayne Dyer
» The Four Agreements by: Don Miguel Ruiz
» A New Earth by: Eckhart Tolle
» Awaken the Giant Within by: Tony Robbins

COMMONLY ASKED QUESTIONS

Q. *I find that I have a blend of imbalances. Several of my balances fall under the Pitta category and several under Vata. What does this mean? What should I focus on?*

A. Great question! This happens a lot. There are multiple layers to the Doshas. An experienced clinician can identify traits where one Dosha can push or block another Dosha. For example Vata can push Pitta. This would act like a windstorm fanning a wild fire causing the fire to spread. From the outside it may look like the fire is the source of the problem, but really it s the blowing of the wind that is making the fire spread and behave in an unruly manner. The rule of thumb is focus on Vata. It is believed that Vata causes the majority of diseases and because we live in a quick, hyper stimulated world (Vata) most of us have a Vata imbalance. By focusing on grounding Vata the other Doshas will come back into alignment. If you have a Ayurveda clinician in your area you may want to have a consultation to learn how the Doshic interplays are affecting you.

Q. *I've had chronic imbalances for as long as I can remember. I've been following all the tools you suggested for over six months now. I'm feeling better but my symptoms are not completely gone yet. Is this normal?*

A. Progress in a positive direction is indicative that you're coming into balance. This is a good thing. Keep it up! If you've had imbalances for years or decades it may take more than several months to get back to 100%. The pace of your improvement will depend of several factors: the strength of the imbalance, the strength of the treatment and the environmental and emotional atmosphere of the patient. In some case, one might feel a drastic shift within days or weeks of apply strategies for balance, in other cases one may need to be more persistent and patient. Seeing an Ayurveda clinician will expedite your alignment because practitioners will likely recognize nuances that we tend to miss when we're self diagnosing and treating.

Q. *All of this has really sparked a deeper interest than I could have ever imagined. What if I wanted to learn more or even be an Ayurveda practitioner myself, where could I go to formally learn Ayurveda.*

A. I love this question! I would love to see Ayurveda as a household name like the practices of yoga, chiropractors, and acupuncture. For that to happen we need more ambassadors. Great schools in the United States include, Kripalu School of Ayurveda in Massachusetts, The Ayurveda Institute in New Mexico, and The California College of Ayurveda among others. The website for NAMA, the National Ayurvedic Medical Association can serve as a directory to explore various avenues. For yoga teachers and holistic practitioners who would like to incorporate Ayurveda into their current scope of work please visit www.ayurveda-orlando.com. I facilitate Ayurveda Training for Yoga Teacher session seasonally.

CPSIA information can be obtained
at www.ICGtesting.com
Printed in the USA
LVHW051141140120
643555LV00004B/105